Advance Praise for *Winn*

"Erudite, insightful, resonant. Stephens's twelve principles go to the heart of what it takes to win any fight."
—Alberto Mella, MBA; speaker; speaking and personal communication coach; Kummooyeh instructor; black belt, Kumdo (Korean fencing)

"A fantastic book! Dr. Stephens's book *Winning Fights* deals with the timeless twelve principles needed for victory in any conflict."
—Andrew Zerling, martial artist; author, *Sumo for Mixed Martial Arts*

"*Winning Fights* is Sun Tzu's *The Art of War* meets Miyamoto Musashi's *The Book of Five Rings*."
—Dr. Craig D. Reid, PhD; martial artist; author, journalist, and martial arts cinema expert

"Holding the world lightweight kickboxing championship for six years straight, you realize you implement these principles naturally. We all knew what we were signing up for, and we called it intestinal fortitude. It is cool to see in print the principles you lived by for so many years!"
—Dale "Sunshine" Frye, former United States lightweight kickboxing champion; two-time world kickboxing champion; movie and television stuntman

"*Winning Fights* is an extremely well-researched book on the strategies and tactics of prevailing in a potentially or actually violent situation.

"I highly recommend this book to anyone interested in fight strategy probing every aspect of a violent encounter and martial history in general."
—David Kahn, US Chief Instructor, Israeli Krav Maga Association; author, *Krav Maga Professional Tactics*

"Awareness can lead to prevention, but in order to be aware, one must first have the knowledge. Dr. Stephens's book outlines some key concepts that would serve as a good base of educating oneself to the path of not just becoming a warrior but a warrior of wisdom."

—Doug Marcaida, Marcaida Kali;
edge impact weapons specialist;
judge, the History Channel's *Forged in Fire*

"In *Winning Fights*, Dr. Phillip Stephens organizes wisdom both ancient and modern into a set of practical principles for approaching and prevailing in a fight, either in or out of a ring."

—Doug Merlino, author, *Beast: Blood, Struggle,
and Dreams at the Heart of Mixed Martial Arts*

"Being a warrior is, in weird part, like being an actor in terms of the better ones are present 100 percent. Dr. Phillip Stephens understands this to his very core and his book hammers this home."

—Eugene S. Robinson, author, *Fight: Everything You Ever
Wanted to Know About Ass-Kicking but Were Afraid
You'd Get Your Ass Kicked for Asking*

"Dr. Stephens covers twelve elements essential to winning a fight. The well-documented concepts he presents put his book among my top reading recommendations."

—George Kirby, judan, Budoshin jujitsu; author, *Jujitsu:
Advanced Techniques for Redirecting an Opponent's Energy*

"We have trained some of the best MMA fighters to ever grace the sport of mixed martial arts. This wonderful book gets really deep into the fighter's mentality and what it takes to survive in such a brutal sport."

—Michael Lyubimov, general manager,
Jackson Wink MMA Academy

"*Winning Fights* truly is a book of principles, and I mean that in important and multiple ways. It is an intelligent book with knowledge gained from centuries of human combat. Highly, highly recommended."

—James Wilson, master rank, kung fu
and full-contact karate/kickboxing; producer,
The Martial Arts Kid and *Paying Mr. McGetty*

"I am a Hollywood stuntman. I've never been able to explain to people the mental-toughness side of my job until I read Dr. Phillip Stephens's book, *Winning Fights*. Whether you have aspirations of becoming a professional fighter, training in martial arts, or boxing as a hobby—or if you have dreams of making any sport your profession—read this book."

—Jeff Jensen, member, Stuntmen's Association of Motion Pictures,
Directors Guild of America, Screen Actors Guild,
The Actor's Studio: Writer/Director Unit,
Hollywood Stuntmen's Hall of Fame

"Jeff Cooper was, and continues to be, legendary in the firearms training world. He spoke and wrote of principles as opposed to techniques. *Winning Fights* addresses the fighting world in a similar fashion."

—Ken Campbell, chief deputy officer, Gunsite Academy, Inc.

"This book is a must-read for anyone serious about fighting. Whether it is for sport or self-preservation, *Winning Fights* breaks down the principles every fighter should learn, understand, and utilize. Cheers to Dr. Stephens for putting these valuable lessons into such a clear, concise, and enjoyable read!"

—Kevin MacDonald, MMA referee; officials trainer for ABC MMA;
Association of Boxing and Combative Sports Commission (ABC);
referee for international UFC and Bellator major promotions

"*Winning Fights* by Dr. Phillip Stephens will stand as a modern classic on management of human conflict in multiple dimensions."

—Massad Ayoob, director, Massad Ayoob Group, LLC;
author of nineteen books, including *Deadly Force in the Gravest Extreme*; chair, Firearms Committee,
American Society of Law Enforcement Trainers

"A fascinating read that covers many facets of MMA."
—Mike Mazzulli, president, Association of Boxing
Commissions and Combative Sports

"*Winning Fights* is a practical and honest guide to all forms of human conflict, whether it is on the battlefield, in the cage, on the mat, or in the boardroom. Drawing on a broad range of sources, Dr. Phillip Stephens shows what it takes to fight and win whatever the form, style, or venue."
—Dr. Peter Maguire, author of *Law and War*,
Facing Death in Cambodia, and *Thai Stick*

"Dr. Phillip Stephens has penned an amazing book covering the strategic implications of martial arts. Not at all a technique book, this is an exploration of the kinds of background development needed to bring any martial art to fruition in the practitioner's life. You will definitely need to read this one several times to take full advantage of Dr. Stephens's enormous contribution."
—Stephen K. Hayes, Black Belt Hall of Fame;
author of twenty-two books

"Enjoy *Winning Fights*, and remember that fighting, while sometimes unavoidable, should be the last rather than the first thing we do in a confrontation."
—Wally Simpson, martial artist;
Chinese-medicine practitioner;
coauthor of *The Encyclopedia of Dim-Mak*

"A handbook about handling conflict from both a physical and philosophical perspective.

"'Finding any semblance of common ground, accepting what comes and dealing with it calmly and dispassionately requires quite a bit of discipline,' Stephens writes in his nonfiction debut, which 'comes from contentment with oneself first.' A strong flavor of Eastern martial culture, reflected in this quote, runs throughout the book, which refers often to such legendary military philosophers as Sun Tzu and the swordsman Miyamoto Musashi (1584–1645), author of *The Book of Five Rings*. But although Stephens spends time talking about spiritual power and mindfulness, the book is predominantly concerned with managing physical violence, either in controlled circumstances, such as a martial arts dojo, or in the chaos of the street. Overall, he's an excellent guide to the realities of such conflict, presenting his principles in clear, sharp prose. Readers who deal regularly with physical altercations—such as war veterans or school guidance counselors—will particularly find a great deal of value in these pages. While outlining twelve crucial elements for securing any kind of victory, Stephens effectively emphasizes core concepts, rather than specific tactics: 'Sure, specialized skill and technique is important,' he writes. 'But it is foundational principles that win any fight regardless of scale or context.' He peppers his text with anecdotes and the examples of a wide array of famous fighters throughout history, from famed actor and martial artist Bruce Lee to Brazilian-jiujitsu fighter Royce Gracie, who was known for 'almost always beating much larger opponents.' Stephens also regularly broadens the backdrop of his study to include large-scale military conflicts, always to illustrate points about the necessity of clear thinking in any kind of fight, and about the economical use of force.

"A clear and strongly worded fighting manual in the long tradition of Sun Tzu."

—*Kirkus Reviews*

WINNING FIGHTS

12 PROVEN PRINCIPLES
FOR WINNING ON THE STREET,
IN THE RING, AT LIFE

Dr. Phillip M. Stephens

YMAA Publication Center, Inc.
Wolfeboro, NH USA

YMAA Publication Center, Inc.
PO Box 480
Wolfeboro, New Hampshire, 03894
1-800-669-8892 • info@ymaa.com • www.ymaa.com

ISBN: 9781594396007 (print) • ISBN: 9781594396014 (ebook)

Managing Editor T. G. LaFredo
Cover design by Axie Breen
This book typeset in Adobe Garamond Pro
Typesetting by Westchester Publishing Services

10 9 8 7 6 5 4 3 2 1

Publisher's Cataloging in Publication

Names: Stephens, Phillip M., author.
Title: Winning fights : 12 principles / Dr. Phillip M. Stephens.
Other titles: 12 proven principles for winning on the street, in the ring, at life.
Description: Wolfeboro, NH USA : YMAA Publication Center, Inc., [2018] |
   Subtitle on cover: 12 proven principles for winning on the street, in the ring,
   at life. | Includes bibliographical references and index.
Identifiers: ISBN: 978-1-59439-600-7 (print) | 978-1-59439-601-4 (ebook) |
   LCCN: 2017961573
Subjects: LCSH: Fighting (Psychology) | Martial arts—Philosophy. | Martial
   arts—Psychological aspects. | Combat—Philosophy. | Combat—Psychological
   aspects. | Boxing—Psychological aspects. | Sports—Psychological aspects. |
   Conflict management—Philosophy. | Negotiation—Psychological aspects. |
   BISAC: SPORTS & RECREATION / Martial Arts & Self-Defense. | SPORTS &
   RECREATION / Sports Psychology. | PSYCHOLOGY / Leadership.
Classification: LCC: BF723.F5 | DDC: 303.6/9—dc23

Printed in Canada

To Wilton M. Stephens,
my late father, who served honorably during the Korean War
(U.S. Air Force staff sergeant).

During my childhood his most frequently used word was
"Honor."

This book is for those who understand its meaning.

TABLE OF CONTENTS

TABLE OF CONTENTS

FOREWORD

by Massad Ayoob

WHEN I MET Dr. Phillip Stephens, it wasn't in the dojo or on the range or in the classroom. It was in the emergency department of a hospital where I was the horizontal patient, with a leg swollen to twice its normal size and a potentially life-threatening blood clot therein. One of the nurses told me reassuringly, "Don't worry, you're getting Dr. Stephens. He's the best there is. He's famous."

The nurse nailed it.

When I walked out of the hospital that night on my own two feet, I knew that I had indeed been treated by a master medical professional. Only later would I know how much else Dr. Stephens had mastered in his highly accomplished life.

By turns a champion fighter in competition and a vastly experienced instructor of others in dojo, ring, and cage, and one of the top medical professionals in his specialty and a role model for others in the same discipline, you are about to find out that Stephens is also a master communicator.

In *Winning Fights*, Dr. Stephens draws from philosophers and kings, from generals and heroic "grunts," from fistfighters and swordfighters and gunfighters, from statecraft and religion and more to clearly delineate universal truths of human conflict.

Deeply researched and up-to-date physiology and psychology figure in Stephens's insightful advice. Certain truths of human conflict are universal, and are equally applicable on the street, on the battlefield, and in wars of words, whether they take place in the courtroom or Debate Society, in a dark alley with no witnesses or on a podium before a vast audience.

Dr. Stephens has fought in the ring against powerful men capable of killing him with a single blow. He has fought disease and trauma countless times, with the trusting patient's life and limb on the line. He has spent his life studying the history and the mind-set of others like himself who fought against sometimes overwhelming odds, in righteous cause. He has prevailed in those endeavors so many times that his thoughts on such things absolutely compel attention.

Human conflict is a vast and multidimensional topic, each subdivision of which can be a life study in and of itself. Phillip Stephens has the education, the experience, and a lifetime of broad-based research to tie those elements together into basic truths that serve across the wide spectrum of arenas in which they take place, often so suddenly that only someone who is prepared for them beforehand will be able to cope, and win.

He understands that a healer of men facing a fast-breaking medical crisis, a General Patton facing Field Marshal Rommel's dreaded Afrika Korps, a petite woman in a dark alley facing a hulking rapist, or a debater in righteous cause squaring off against a silver-tongued devil will all need the same resolve, preparedness, determination, and wherewithal to bring the conflict to a just conclusion.

And, most important, he shares the tools, the formulae, that have been proven to prevail in such circumstances.

Perhaps the greatest value in *Winning Fights* is that it applies to a wide range of stages upon which conflict takes place. In four-and-a-half decades of working within the justice system and teaching people how to win fights, I've learned that you can be wearing a hat that says "Defensive Tactics Coach," "Shooting Coach," or even the currently popular "Life Coach" and find yourself recommending the exact same strategies and tactics. It's about principle, not technique.

It has been an honor to write this foreword for Dr. Stephens's book, and I hope you benefit from his wisdom as much as I have.

ACKNOWLEDGMENTS

AIRARD FITZ STEPHEN was the eleventh-century commander of William the Conqueror's ship, the *Mora*. It seems fitting for his great-grandson to write a book on fighting. Though he died in battle, I'm thankful he lived long enough to have children.

The Stephens family crest motto is *Consilio et armis*, which means "by wisdom and arms." An expert in heraldry has translated this as "we can talk or we can fight." This motto exemplifies the spirit of this work.

Nobody has been more important to me in the pursuit of this project than my wife, Gina, and sons, Matthew and Andrew. They patiently traveled with me to countless martial arts tournaments across the United States, missing holidays and celebrating birthdays in strange cities. They continually support my writing.

I'm indebted to the experience and training I received from Master Nathaniel Thompson and Master Johnny Miller, who trained me for two world championships and other martial arts titles. I am also grateful for the continued support of my black belt brothers, especially those at Dojo Knights mentioned in this work.

I especially appreciate the valuable feedback from unnamed members of the U.S. Marines and U.S. Army Third Special Forces Group, stationed at Fort Bragg, North Carolina. One person whose name is not classified

ACKNOWLEDGMENTS

information is my friend Frank Trenery, a retired marine and fellow martial artist who inspired the chapter on timing.

The North Carolina Boxing Commission, and specifically Agent Terrance Merriweather, a U.S. Army veteran, was especially supportive, as were the Alcohol Law Enforcement agents who work for the Commission covering fighting events across the state.

Retired North Carolina Highway Patrol Captain Randy Hammonds provided a living example of leadership.

The illustrator is Roger Musashi Reeder, a colleague from Japan. His handwritten kanji adds authentic and beautiful value.

The reviewers are especially appreciated, all of whom are experts in their field. I extend my heartfelt thanks to each of them for their input. I am humbled by their willingness to be a part of the book.

I am thankful to the professionals at YMAA Publishing. They bring the best out of authors. Their input is amazing, and many there touched this project. After the words were written, they were the ones who helped breathe life into the work.

Finally, writing something like this would not have been possible without a supportive mother and a father who inspired me from a young age to understand character, the warrior spirit, and the meaning of honor.

My prayer is for this work to stand the test of time; it is not the culmination of my thoughts alone, but the wisdom of over two thousand years.

INTRODUCTION

Winning fights is based on principles—not techniques.

TECHNIQUE IS IMPORTANT. But techniques change, adapt, and evolve. Principles are timeless. Bruce Lee recognized this truth, and advised to "absorb what is useful, discard what is useless and add what is specifically your own."[1] To Lee, there was no single superior style of fighting. He even referred to his methods as the "style of no style."

All fighters face the same challenges. Whether just two people fighting in a ring for sport or two armies engaged in geopolitical conflict, a fight is a fight.

Eastern and Western military strategists throughout millennia have agreed on the principles that overcome the challenges faced during a fight, whether between individuals or nations. The basic principles for winning fights simply do not change and are like laws of nature ignored at one's peril. But the knowledge is often lost in the noise of literature or the static of techniques, tactics, and form. The average fighter then loses sight of these foundational principles, which are required to win and must be applied before any other strategy.

Winning fights, surviving conflict, and successfully engaging in combat rely on these principles. Specialized skill and technique are important, but it is foundational principles that win any fight regardless of scale or context. Basic principles are essentially laws that govern the success of survival from personal to global conflicts.

These same principles have many parallels and applications in life and business affairs. If these principles are understood and a warrior code is adhered to on a daily basis, the success of winning fights will spill over into successful peaceful routine activities as well. Societies would be more polite and fewer fights would be fought. Why is it important for a peaceful person to understand these principles? A classic Eastern saying is that, "It is better to be a warrior in a garden, than a gardener in a war."[2]

Peace and violence are not mutually exclusive concepts. All warriors want peace. In fact, warriors who have seen violence especially want peace. But history has demonstrated that peace can be elusive. Preparing for conflict is the best way to ensure peace.

Knowing how to win a fight isn't in opposition to peace or love. It is a part of peace and love. If you want peace then you must be willing to fight for it. You must be willing to defend the people you love. Warriors pray for peace but are willing to stand against evil in the world. Violent men with discipline are the only ones who stand between the world and evil.

This book is not about style. It is about concepts that are necessary for winning and are perilous to ignore, as evidenced by thousands of years of trial and error. It is the culmination of the work of the greatest martial strategists in history.

Martial artists have argued for centuries about which fighting style has the most effective techniques. Lee was the first modern-day martial artist to emphasize principle over technique, as principles of winning are timeless and are not confined by style. Winning is embodied by philosophy and strategy. This is why a work on principle rather than simply technique is important.

More than two thousand years ago (c. 5th century BCE), Chinese General Sun Tzu wrote one of the oldest known works concerning foundational principles for winning fights. The Art of War presented a time-tested philosophy for winning wars, managing conflict, and leading organizations.[3] There are other ancient military texts similar to Sun Tzu's work, including The Book of Five Rings, by Miyamoto Musashi, Hagakure, by Yamamoto Tsunetomo, and On War,[4] by Carl Van Clausewitz. Sun Tzu's work is the most prominent and earliest example, but all of these compositions echo similar principles, as truth is truth evidenced by similar themes for winning. Time, technology, and even context have had little impact on these principles, which have been echoed countless times in works spanning two thousand years.

Many of these early texts formed the foundation for modern military theory and have survived the test of time and conflict. They devote chapters to broad aspects of warfare and focus on principle, strategy, philosophy, and mind-set. So even these early texts on warfare agree on the foundational principles of winning fights regardless of the techniques or tools employed to win those fights.

Several years after the death of Bruce Lee, who popularized martial arts in the West, Lt. Col. Jeff Cooper, a former Marine who served in World War II and the Korean War, founded the American Pistol Institute (later called Gunsite Academy).[5] While Bruce Lee was best known for his development of unarmed approaches to winning fights, Cooper taught the pragmatic use of firearms. Most shooting fundamentals can be traced back to the work of Cooper, who many consider to be the creator of modern-day handgun shooting techniques.

But like Bruce Lee, Cooper recognized the importance of principle over technique. He felt that neither weapons nor martial art skills were the most important means of surviving a lethal confrontation. To Cooper, the primary tool was mind-set.[6] He articulated these basic principles often in his shooting lessons, just as Bruce Lee and Sun Tzu had done. These modern fighters reconfirmed that fighting principles were consistent and timeless.

On November 12, 1993, the first Ultimate Fighting Championship (UFC) aired from the McNichols Sports Arena in Denver, Colorado.[7] During those early fights there were no weight classes or judges. There also were only two rules: no biting and no eye gouging. Matches ended by submission, knockout, or one of the fighters' corners throwing in the towel. Gloves were permitted but mostly for the protection of the fighters' hands, not the other way around.

Royce Gracie won UFC 1, UFC 2, and UFC 4. He fought to a draw in UFC 5. Gracie popularized Brazilian jujutsu and almost always conquered much larger opponents.[8] The Gracie brand of jujutsu had a significant impact on the UFC, which continued to grow and was soon followed by other successful organizations, such as Bellator. The principles of how a smaller fighter could successfully defeat a much larger opponent are at the heart of the Gracie system, which descended from ancient Japanese warriors. It was put on full display during these fights and subsequently changed Western thinking about how fights are won.

To pardon the pun, fighters are still grappling today with what will be successful in winning fights in a competition involving few rules. The ground fighting techniques of Gracie are now well known and practiced by many. The principles that successful fighters apply to their craft set them apart. Certainly, Gracie's techniques helped him to win fights, but the principles and mind-set that he employed were equally important. A fighter can't expect to enter a contest against a much larger opponent armed with technique alone.

These principles work on any scale and transcend fighting, and I believe they are now more important than ever. My father served in the U.S. Strategic Air Command during the Korean War. Their mission was one of deterrence, and its success is evidenced by the fact that we avoided nuclear war. It was a classic Sun Tzu strategy of subduing an enemy without fighting; a show of force can result in peace. Few appreciate the success of U.S. strength during the Cold War and the strategies that kept us safe. It's tough to appreciate avoiding a fight through strength because there is nothing to measure except the lack of a fight.

Let's face it, humans are a violent species. What's worse is that many enemies are not deterred by the possibility of a nuclear exchange and actually may have an apocalyptic mission. Some strategists think it is better to simply fight and win than to employ deterrence strategies against an enemy that has nothing to lose. Totally winning a fight is more important than ever in a world where nothing will deter the enemy. Winning is the only option.

Every fighter must understand the fundamental principles that are required for winning a fight if a fight is inevitable. These principles are universal and apply whether the conflict is on the battlefield or in a dark alley. Quite simply, they are the principles of war and apply to the modern-day warrior armed with the latest technology just as they did to a Samurai armed with a sword. A fight is still a personal thing. Its sting hasn't dulled over time and the edge of the warriors' weapons is still intact. If anything, weapons have become sharper.

THE 12 PRINCIPLES

Readers may well ask, why just 12 principles? Well, there are numerous principles found in historical and modern texts, many of which overlap or are emphasized differently. Initially, I tried to encapsulate the history of fighting into 10 principles to make it simpler.

I have studied and taught martial arts and have won a couple of world tournament titles in the self-defense division, along with a bunch of smaller ones. I even help write the rules on fighting as a member of the Boxing Commission.

I also have a doctorate in Health Science (DHSc) and approach the study of the ancient texts from an academic point of view as someone who teaches evidence-based solutions and critical thought. Someone with this experience should be able to fit the concepts into a concise framework to make them easier to study, comprehend, and apply.

In my research, I polled some combat personnel with whom I worked and others stationed at Fort Bragg in North Carolina, home to the U.S. Army Special Operations Command. This put things into perspective. The experiences of these heroes dwarfed my fighting knowledge. My study of fighting was scholarly and my practice was in controlled environments. These guys live or die by the warrior spirit and view the principles from a different perspective.

Nothing compares to talking to a guy about fighting who has been shot at many times. These modern-day warriors enriched my knowledge of fighting. My academic approach and martial arts experience were enhanced by my interactions with these heroes, whose lives depend on the proper application of these principles. I found that training was good and academic knowledge was necessary, but writing about fighting isn't complete without the added perspective of someone who has repeatedly applied them to survive.

My work with the SFOs led to the addition of two principles: timing and fortitude. "Timing" was first suggested by a U.S. Marine and "fortitude" was seen as being of paramount importance by many in the field. Specifically, members of the 3rd Special Forces Group (Airborne) provided feedback. With multiple tours of duty in Iraq and Afghanistan over many branches of service, these silent warriors provided invaluable insight that was practical and revealed the true heart of the fighting spirit. Their input complemented the academic approach to the material. These chapters on timing and fortitude amplify the basic principles explored in the first 10 chapters.

The last four chapters explore how tactics, weapons, honor, and words factor into fighting. These sections grew from my research. Tactics are examples of practical application of the principles. Weapons are an essential extension of a fighter. Honor is especially important, as it was vital to the success of ancient societies. Words have long been the first weapon drawn in conflict. My analysis of fighting with words was another addition that emerged from those interviews. These last four sections are intended to add value to the main principles.

The 12 principles that provide the framework for this book sometimes overlap. There are also crucial secondary principles within each principle. However, the 12 items encapsulate the theme of what it takes to win a fight.

Technology may change. Techniques may change. What man fights about may change. But the principles that win fights remain the same, as does the heart of a warrior, which is required to apply these principles.

These 12 principles were forged by history and have been researched with academic rigor and continually practiced by warriors throughout the ages.

Notes

1. Bruce Lee, *The Tao of Jeet Kune Do* (Santa Clarita, CA: Ohara, 1975).
2. Alberto Mella, "The Warrior in the Garden" (The Gentlemen's Brotherhood, 2017), www.thegentlemensbrotherhood.com/inspiration/the-warrior-in-the -garden/.
3. Sun Tzu, *The Art of War and Other Classics of Eastern Thought* (New York: Barnes & Noble, 2013).
4. Miyamoto Musashi, *The Five Rings, Miyamoto Musashi's Art of Strategy: The New Illustrated Edition of the Japanese Warrior Classic* (New York: Quarto

Publishing Group, 2012); Yamamoto Tsunetomo, *Hagakure* (New York: Kodansha International, 1983); Carl Von Clausewitz, *On War* (New York: Barnes & Noble, 2004).

5. Jeff Cooper, "About Us" (Paulden, AZ: Gunsite Academy, 1976), https://www.gunsite.com/about-us/.

6. Brad Fitzpatrick, "Col. Jeff Cooper: Developing a Defensive Mindset," *Guns & Ammo* (2015), www.gunsandammo.com/personal-defense/col-jeff-cooper-developing-a-defensive-mindset/.

7. Joe Nguyen, "UFC 1 Took Place in Denver on Nov. 12, 1993," *Denver Post,* November 12, 1993, blogs.denverpost.com/sports/2015/11/12/tbt-ufc-1-took-place-in-denver-on-nov-12-1993/28298/.

8. "About Royce" (2015), roycegracie.com/about-royce/.

SECTION 1: TWELVE PRINCIPLES

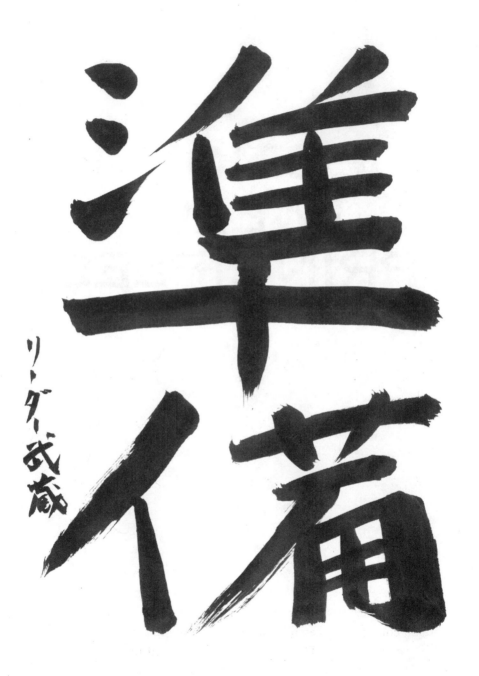

PREPARATION

PREPARATION HAS BEEN one of the primary principles for winning fights since the beginning of recorded time. It is a universal principle that applies to everything from individual encounters to wars. The concept is self-evident. It has survived the test of time and is a good place to start.

From a tactical standpoint, the first principle should be surprise. However, the element of surprise is often afforded to the attacker and is primarily a function of offensive action. We will discuss how to introduce surprise defensively a bit later. But preparation helps counter surprise, so again, it's a good place to start.

In general, average citizens simply react to an aggressor, and thus relinquish the element of surprise. But preparation helps minimize any surprises that might benefit an opponent. The first principle is simply to be prepared for conflict. This principle is historically important.

Over two thousand years ago, Chinese General Sun Tzu foresaw who would win or lose a battle based on the extent of each general's preparation.[1] More recently, former president Ronald Reagan noted this truth in quoting George Washington, who said that to be prepared for war is one of the most effective means of preserving peace.[2]

This concept reaches biblical proportions. King Solomon relates in Christian scripture: "The prudent see danger and take refuge, but the simple keep going and pay the penalty" (Proverbs 22:3). In the New

Living Translation, taking "refuge" is to "take precautions" or, in other words, to be prepared. This ancient wisdom from Sun Tzu to King Solomon is clearly applicable to modern-day warriors. Preparation is vital and involves more than physical preparation.

Former Ultimate Fighting Championship (UFC) heavyweight champion Randy Couture once said that a fight is 90 percent mental and only 10 percent physical. Yet most fighters train 90 percent physical and 10 percent mental.[3]

Ronda Rousey is a more recent mixed martial arts competitor and judo Olympian. Her preparation made her the most dominant male or female athlete in sports. Rousey recalled a story of breaking her toe during training when she was a teenager. Rather than pampering Rousey, her mother, a judo champion in her own right, made her run laps. Her mother later told her that the reason she pushed Rousey to continue despite a broken toe was to demonstrate to her that she could do it. Rousey developed a "never quit" attitude, and this preparation established her foundation as a champion.[4]

Rousey embodied this principle, especially in early fights. Her preparation was always structured and meticulous. She embodied other principles as well, which combined to make a champion. But while her preparation seemed principled in UFC 207 against Amanda Nunes,[5] the result is a cautionary tale of how no principle stands alone.

Rousey, who is an expert grappler, was up against a boxer and lost early in the match during moments when blows were being exchanged. Now no one expects every fighter to be indomitable in every fight or to demonstrate perfect examples of every principle in every moment over the course of a career. We also don't know what every fighter had planned or was thinking. A million plans can go wrong between preparation and execution. Sometimes a brief moment of miscalculation or an instant of opportunity is all it takes to win or lose a fight. Nevertheless, history will record that Rousey was ultimately a winner who paved the way for women in the world of fighting arts and was one of the most competitive athletes of all time.

As head basketball coach for the University of South Carolina, Frank Martin was being interviewed after winning some important games.

Martin was a tough coach and explained his philosophy to the reporter, "We've gotten to the place in society to where we think that we're supposed to make things easy for kids and then when they fail as men, we blame them."[6] He went on to explain that he demands his players work hard because success is not an easy thing. Martin believes kids haven't changed. Adults have changed, and demand less of kids instead of preparing them for what life is truly about.

Preparation involves both mental and physical elements, with mental preparation being the most important. It can be a tough thing. But it is the foremost concern in preparing for any fight whether the encounter is for sport, self-defense, or war.

How you prepare will be determined by a myriad of factors. Size, gender, where someone lives, training, access or familiarity with weapons all determine how someone physically responds to violence and where to start in preparing for such encounters. If the preparation is training for a sport, the answer is much easier as the environment in these encounters is fairly controlled and the subsequent actions are predictable. Therefore, you have an awareness of exactly how to prepare, as all the variables are known in advance of the conflict. Sports have boundaries and rules.

How you prepare depends on who the enemy is and where the battle will be waged. In the fourth century BCE, Sun Tzu referred to knowing the enemy as a vital strategy in warfare.[7] Regardless of whether the fight is organized sport or a fight for life, knowing yourself and the opponent is essential preparation. Ask Rousey or any successful fighter who always prepares well, but in retrospect may have prepared differently for fights they lost.

In a confined sports arena with rules, these elements are controlled and the enemy is clearly known. But outside a controlled environment confrontations are less predictable. This simply means that in preparing for sport, self-defense, or war, the only difference is the degree of predictability and control over the encounter.

At the other extreme of conflict, war has no rules. While technically there are some rules of engagement, there is a saying among warriors that if you find yourself in a fair fight your tactics suck. So preparation must occur whether for sport or war with these parameters in mind.

Again, this affects only about 10 percent of your preparation in terms of evaluating your physical strengths, weaknesses, the level of your training, and whether you live in or travel to a dangerous area and are more likely to encounter violence. The remaining 90 percent of preparation is mental. Sun Tzu called this knowing oneself, which is as important as knowing your enemy. It's Ronda Rousey knowing she can fight even with a broken toe. She says pain is just information. It's the Navy Seals "never-give-up" attitude. Each individual Seal isn't necessarily the very best fighter. What sets them apart is that Seals are so mentally tough that they will keep fighting regardless of how many times they are knocked down. It is a mental toughness shared by many Special Operators.

Sun Tzu, Rousey, and Navy Seals understand pushing beyond physical limitations. We discuss fortitude later, but knowing mental limits is important. Good fighters prepare in order to know these limits. A fighter doesn't want to learn his limits during a fight. Good preparation helps push those limits higher with this first principle impacting the last.

Bruce Lee was a great martial artist and spoke often regarding the process of self-cultivation. Both ancient and modern warriors recognize that mental preparation must occur first and foremost. The inner battle must be won before attempting to prevail in any external battle.

If you size up your physical preparation and have an idea of who your enemy might be and prepare accordingly—how do you size yourself up? This answer is also found in ancient wisdom.

Japanese military strategists often reflected the Chinese Taoist concepts of Wu-Sing, or the Five Elements of earth, air, water, fire, and void, as the Gojo-Goyoku.[8] They applied these concepts to the mind as five feelings or weaknesses. This was part of the black art of the Ninja who utilized the five weaknesses to defeat an enemy:

1. Fear
2. Lust
3. Anger
4. Greed
5. Sympathy

Though these feelings or emotions change dynamically there is always one that dominates. Understanding the weaknesses that dominate yourself and your opponent is vital to winning. A fighter must overcome personal weakness while exploiting the weakness of an opponent.

For example, sympathy may be a weakness in a pacifist who abhors violence. This sympathy creates an internal conflict, as the individual is not mentally prepared to harm others even if under threat. This is a serious limitation that can be exploited by a violent person.

Usually, anger overcomes sympathy. Someone wishing to harm the children of even a passive mother will cultivate the mother's anger. Any sympathy she may have for the attacker will immediately disappear as she directs her anger toward the attacker in order to protect her children. This is the balance of emotions that occur and manifest themselves as either strengths or weaknesses.

Fear is the most common weakness a fighter must overcome. Though anger can overcome fear, it too must be under control. Uncontrolled anger results in recklessness, and uncontrolled fear can be paralyzing.

The basic internal preparation for controlling fear is recognizing it is perceptual. It is not something a fighter overcomes as it can be controlled much like anger. Like anger, fear can be focused to good use.

Nelson Mandela said that courage wasn't the absence of fear but the triumph over it.[9] Plato described courage as knowing what not to fear.[10] The point being that fear has its place and is a natural response to perceived threats. It simply needs to be focused so that it doesn't become irrational and result in paralysis of action. Understanding internal weaknesses and the opposing motivation to overcome that weakness is vital to mindful preparation.

Firearms instructors advise students that if they are not prepared to utilize their weapon to kill someone in the event their life is threatened, then they probably should not be carrying a weapon. Carrying a weapon is one thing. Mentally knowing you are prepared to use it is quite another. If someone carrying a weapon isn't prepared to use it, then they may be bringing a weapon for their attacker to use against them. Being prepared is understanding individual weaknesses and mentally overcoming those weaknesses.

Men perish for lack of vision is an old proverb. A winning attitude that overcomes weaknesses is vital to good preparation and creates a winning vision. Science supports this ancient proverb as you must first see yourself winning.

VISUALIZATION

There is a story about an American prisoner of war in Vietnam who for seven years was isolated from others and had little physical activity in confinement. However, during his entire time in captivity he visualized himself playing golf at his favorite courses every day. He imagined himself dressed in golf clothes. He included every detail of the experience in his mind down to the fragrance of the trees and how he gripped the club. He pictured each ball rolling across the green.

He was in no hurry. He was in captivity and not going anywhere. So he mentally played golf. Upon his release, he returned home and when he played golf for real the first time his game had actually improved.[11]

Regardless of how true the story was, it has been confirmed by research. Studies with athletes including Olympians have concluded that visualization techniques aid performance improvement. Visualization is now an accepted training technique and a part of sports science, as there is a powerful relationship between mental and physical performance. It is a useful preparation tool.

Research has demonstrated that brain activity patterns among weight lifters were the same whether the weight lifter actually lifted a large weight or simply imagined it.[12] This is remarkable knowledge. The brain doesn't differentiate signaling for thought and signaling for action in terms of areas activated by the brain. Whether we are conducting the action or not, it still enhances the same area of the brain.

A study by Ranganathan et al., "From Mental Power to Muscle Power—Gaining Strength by Using the Mind," even revealed that mental practice was almost as effective as physical practice.[13] Furthermore, doing both was more effective than doing either alone. Specifically, those who went to the gym had a 30 percent muscle increase. Those who conducted mental exercise were able to experience a 13.5 percent increase. Mental visualization alone achieved nearly half the increase as physical application. This is the power of thought.

Thoughts simply produce the same mental instructions as action. The key is engaging as many of the senses as possible during visualization practice. Emotions, smells, sights, hearing, and the environment that is visualized are all important. Walt Disney reportedly said, "If you can dream it, you can do it." (The quote was actually written by Imagineer Tom Fitzgerald at Disney.)[14] His view was literally visionary, as the power of visualization is greater than imagined decades ago as it relates to physical performance.

Understand that violent encounters are possible. Visualize violent encounters that may occur. Then mentally and physically prepare your actions. Have a vision for what you will do. This preparation has value.

Most people have no idea what they would do when faced with violence let alone prepare through visualization. They have never thought about it. Therefore they never train for it. They never prepare. When confronted with violence, they perish for lack of vision. This lack of mental preparation results in paralysis of action, which may lead to deadly consequences.

RECOGNITION

Mindful recognition of hostility is important. If you recognize conflict, know your enemies regarding where conflict will originate, and understand when violence is escalating, then you will be prepared to stop violence sometimes before it even begins. After all, the best way to win a fight is to avoid one. The best way to start preparing for violence is to imagine what you would do if violence were encountered. Thoughts occur before action as nothing happens without a thought.

An approaching stranger asking for a cigarette may seem innocent. But often this may be a ruse for a predator to get closer to his prey. An acquaintance may suggest a private meeting somewhere. This may be innocent as well. But if either subtle act seems out of context, both could be precursors to violence. Mental preparation for these encounters is important as well as recognizing patterns of behavior that just don't fit the context.

ANTICIPATE

A friend returning from a war zone related that one of the primary means of survival was to constantly discern friend from foe before anyone was allowed to approach the troops. They didn't obsess over it, but they were always mentally prepared for conflict at every turn and incorporated constant preparedness in their daily routine.

This may seem paranoid. But preparation means controlling how close someone gets to you and preparing for potential conflict, even during seemingly ordinary circumstances that are part of your daily routine. It is these innocent encounters that often escalate quickly and paralyze those who fail to prepare for the escalation of an innocent encounter. Controlling your environment does have its limitations. But being able to control more space around you affords you more safety. Verbal and non-verbal communication of boundaries is important. Anticipate violence from anyone who crosses these boundaries.

It is the ability to be alert that helps counter the element of surprise afforded to aggressors. Preparation helps mitigate the paralysis of action that occurs with sudden violence. Being aware is another principle discussed later. But one must prepare first in order to develop the skill of awareness.

MENTAL EDGE

Mental preparation combats the initial shock and inaction that accompanies the first moments of unexpected conflict. Mindful preparation of knowing the potential enemy and understanding what to do in the event the enemy strikes help maintain the presence of mind needed to overcome conflict.

There are basically three ways to mentally foreshadow and survive violence:

1. Avoid it entirely.
2. Escape if it can't be avoided.
3. Devastate the attacker's ability to fight if escape is not possible.

Avoiding and escaping require presence of mind. So again, two out of three methods to survive violence are mental. Both involve being prepared with a plan and being alert in order to execute a plan.

This is consistent with the discussed concept that preparation for a fight is 90 percent mental and 10 percent physical—ultimately, winning a fight requires a prepared mind. In many circumstances, if conflict is avoided or escape is achieved, the fight is considered won as much as if the enemy had been physically defeated. The old adage that the best way to win a fight is to not be involved in one is true.

A quick caveat is that if avoiding a fight will simply escalate into a worse conflict later, then a quick end is usually the best strategy. This is assuming the conflict is inevitable, meaning escape or avoidance is impossible. Avoidance simply postpones the outcome in these instances. The fight will happen sooner or later and it is best fought on your terms at a time of your choosing. But that's if the situation involves planned conflict such as wars, though it could be personal such as occurs with bullies or other ongoing conflict in which the aggressor simply isn't going to allow you to escape. If the fight is inevitable, fight it on your terms—not theirs.

Master Johnny Miller is an old school martial artist who trained me for two world championships. He would relate this concept of ending an inevitable fight before it escalated further by humorously quoting his own instructor, a Vietnam veteran, with the tongue-in-cheek quip, "If you owe a man something, whether it's $20 or a butt whooping—pay him." Though related in jest it placed inevitable fights in the same context as a debt to be settled but settled on the fighter's terms, not the opponent's. Never fight a fight at the time, place, or rules chosen by the opposition.

Violent Reality

There are violent people in this world who do not care if you are peaceful. They do not care about your religious beliefs, political views, or even you as a person. They have no regard for civility. Some have mental disorders and are simply crazy.

Motives for violence vary. Some aggressors may be criminals. They may be mentally unstable, irrational, or just evil. Ultimately, your views on violence do not affect their actions as dark forces drive them. You must understand this, as there sometimes is no rational explanation for the violence committed by many individuals. There are psychopaths and other depraved individuals in the world for whom normal laws of human emotion, reasoning, and interaction do not apply.

In fact, some researchers believe that 1 in every 100 men is born a clinical psychopath and 1 in every 300 women.[15] Women have a lower incidence of the disorder. Despite the emotional deficiency, many psychopaths and other categories of individuals with personality disorders learn to mimic normal emotion to otherwise fit into society. In some cases there is no rational explanation for violent behavior. And it is sometimes difficult to differentiate these individuals from the rest of the populace.

Millions of victims learn this truth the hard way. You can either be an unprepared victim or make violent encounters impractical for the perpetrator. Making violent encounters impractical for the perpetrator is the solution to violence. No law or other solution supersedes this truth.

Exposing the mind to this understanding is vital preparation and reprograms the brain to respond to conflict. If the mind is prepared for conflict, then it will become less chaotic during real battle so that paralysis of action or the fog of war will be minimized. In many ways, the mind must not only be constantly aware that conflict can occur but when it occurs the mind must achieve a certain level of detachment from the very violence for which it is prepared.

Mental Detachment

Many studies, such as a 2007 Dutch study among military police,[16] demonstrate that emotional dissonance mediates psychological strain within the emotional demands of the job. A 2006 study among jobs expected to exhibit a certain degree of emotional detachment such as police officers and nurses had earlier identified emotional dissonance as not only a coping factor but there was a cost in terms of burnout as well.[17] Mental detachment is a double-edged sword.

In other words, the studies expect those in high-stress jobs to form some mental detachment from the trauma they witness daily. Researchers wanted to know if this detachment is helpful or harmful. In the short term it seems to be helpful. If there is prolonged exposure to trauma requiring this coping mechanism then it can lead to long-term consequences such as burnout.

"Cognitive dissonance" is the term used to describe the uncomfortable tension between conflicting thoughts and actions. Sometimes, cognitive dissonance occurs unconsciously. Purposeful cognitive dissonance internally protects the mind from unpleasant environments. Cognitive dissonance simply makes the mind comfortable during uncomfortable situations. This disassociation is complex and has both positive and negative effects. This is why morbid humor among professionals in high-stress environments serves a useful purpose. Laughing about the risk of death or the horror that surrounds them is a useful coping mechanism.

The point here is professional soldiers and others engaged in violent or unpleasant environments use cognitive dissonance to their advantage. Fighters learn how to disassociate from the violence they are engaged in for the same reasons as police officers or nurses disassociate from the daily horror they may witness.

This is one reason that moral codes of honor are important. Warrior codes are discussed at length here because without them this mental disassociation from violence doesn't work well. If a fighter feels nothing after delivering extreme violence toward another human being then this is suggestive of sociopathy. Moral codes and cognitive disassociation provide these mental protections and justifications for violence.

Psychiatrist Jonathan Shay is an expert on combat trauma. In his 1994 book, *Achilles in Vietnam*, he writes that "When a leader destroys the legitimacy of the army's moral order by betraying 'what's right,' he inflicts manifold injuries on his men."[18] If a fighter has a high moral ground for the violence he is inflicting, there is less guilt afterward.

Fighters must deliver overwhelming violence to win. Because they are not sociopaths yet must deliver sociopathic-level violence to stop sociopaths, there must be delineating factors and support structures. If these mental tools are not in place the fighter may be reluctant to deliver the necessary violence to win or may deliver the violence but be unprepared for the mental aftermath of anguish and guilt that may occur even with preparation. This is why honor codes and warrior ethics are more than just philosophy. They are real tools for fighting. Warrior traditions of brotherhood are more than just testosterone-filled traditions. They have purposeful value.

Mental preparation is vital to understand what is needed to win a life-or-death fight. A moral warrior code of ethics and honor is what separates the warrior from a thug and is a necessary component of this preparation. Strong faith with supportive friends and family are stable support systems to overcome the aftermath of violence. Being thoughtful about the consequences of violent conflict in advance helps mitigate the barriers to doing what is necessary to win and coping with the aftereffects.

PHYSICAL PREPARATION

Physical preparation is also vital. Master Rick Campbell and Tim Bryant are fellow black belts who prepare students vigorously before every class. Warm-up exercises of 750 jumping jacks or hundreds of sit-ups before class is not unusual. Their purpose is fitness before even beginning lessons on self-defense.

When a student asked if this amount of physical preparation was overkill, Master Campbell's response was that if faced with two attackers there will be two sets of lungs opposing the students' one set. Master Campbell wants them to be as prepared as possible. If the student can't do 750 jumping jacks, he should do as many as possible, pushing his limits. Why do 50 jumping jacks when the student could do 100? Why do 100 when the student could really do 200? His point is that everyone should keep pushing to achieve his or her maximum potential. Physical limits must be known and a safe dojo is the place to test those limits. A fighter should never give up or quit.

This is what sets black belts apart from other martial artists. Black belts are not supermen guaranteed to win every time just because they are black belts. But you can be assured they will keep getting up, dusting themselves off, and continuing to fight as long as possible. Black belts aren't going to quit. It's a black belt mentality.

The most successful fighters train as they wish to fight—sometimes harder. The wisdom is that it is better to cry in training and laugh on the battlefield. The more bruises a fighter receives in training, the fewer he receives in real combat.

Understanding the principles of winning fights is the beginning of preparation for violent encounters. Studying martial arts on some level is another step in preparation or otherwise training to utilize weapons in some fashion. But understand it isn't a certain technique, weapon, or style of martial art that adequately prepares someone for a fight. There are many organized systems of training and differing fight methodologies. The important aspect is finding what fits you and what applies to the real world irrespective of styles, belt rankings, tournaments, or whatever other reason there is to study martial arts.

If you are studying for fitness, then there are many programs that fill that need. If your goal is internal reflection, there are many excellent internal martial arts to explore. But if it is for real-world self-defense, then you must filter out what does not fill that need and focus on what is tactically useful. Before entering a martial arts class, everyone should first determine why they want to study martial arts.

TRAINING

Classical training has failed many practitioners when confronted with real violence. Again, they trained physically in controlled environments but their mental preparation and physical application of skill was limited. They simply weren't prepared for the chaos and sheer violence in a real fight. Their training in a controlled environment could not translate to the chaotic violence outside of an air-conditioned training hall. Whether a given art has a practical application is an ongoing discussion in the martial arts community. But that isn't the right question. The correct question is why the person wishes to train.

Some may want the skills transferable to the streets. But others may simply want exercise or to study the classics. Students shouldn't fool themselves by taking a martial art class for one reason—thinking it will be the answer for all conflict outside the gym. Why you choose to study will answer the question of what to study.

What you study, how you train, and whether you carry a weapon must be decided ahead of time depending on your mind-set and level of exposure to violence. Decide how you will defend yourself then seek appropriate preparation. Prevailing laws may even dictate how people can defend themselves if confronted with aggression.

Sadly, if a law-abiding citizen is in an area that forbids carrying weapons, then the level of protection afforded to being in that area is already decided by someone else. The criminal element typically doesn't follow laws. Assault, robbery, and such are already illegal. Just making it unlawful doesn't mean everyone will obey those laws. Ultimately, you are responsible for your own self-preservation and for those you love. But you must also obey the law and this is part of preparation regarding how you can protect yourself depending on where you travel.

Learning a martial art, taking a self-defense class, obtaining concealed weapons training or other knowledge-based preparation is up to the individual and is best decided in advance of violence.

MIND-SET

Study how people act and move around you. Prepare for how you will react if someone attempts to breach your personal space. Develop a mindset of self-defense. Those who are not prepared will appear weak and attract predators. Those who are prepared typically manifest this preparation through confidence. Conflict is often avoided by simple preparation and thought process.

Miyamoto Musashi was a Samurai warrior of great renown who lived in the sixteenth century. He is the author of the still-popular *Book of Five Rings*, an ancient text on fighting strategy, tactics, and philosophy.[19]

Legend has it that he never lost a fight. He killed as many as 25 men in duels before age 21 and well over 60 in his lifetime.[20] This is not counting his many victories in larger battles. He clearly was the most skilled swordsman of his day, but there is one account of him winning without fighting.[21]

There are many versions of the story and some attribute the hero of the story as being Tsukahara Bokuden rather than Musashi.[22] Some accounts say it was a young, impetuous Samurai who challenged our hero Musashi to a duel to prove himself. In other accounts, a drunk bothered Musashi by challenging him to a fight as Musashi tried to sleep in a boat.

Whether a young inexperienced Samurai or a drunk, in each account neither was a match for Musashi. But Musashi agreed to the duel stating they must go to a remote island nearby to avoid tipping the boat over.

Musashi rowed toward the island with the angry young challenger aboard. Anger grew in the young warrior, who was anxious to prove himself. Musashi calmly rowed closer and closer to the island. The young man asked Musashi what style of swordsmanship he practiced. Without looking at the young hothead, Musashi replied that he practiced the art of fighting without fighting. This angered the young Samurai even more as he thought he was being insulted.

Once the boat touched the shore the challenger immediately jumped off the boat, anxious to duel. But as the challenger turned to face Musashi with his hand on his sword and his feet in the water, all he saw was Musashi rowing away from the shore, leaving the challenger on the remote island. If this story sounds familiar, it is because Bruce Lee adapted it for a scene in the film *Enter the Dragon*.

The story does not say why Musashi decided to spare this particular challenger. Musashi was known for being a bit unorthodox and not caring as much for formal protocol as he was defeating his opponent. His success supports adherence to these principles as vital to winning. But in this instance he wisely won the fight without fighting, sparing the youthful hothead's life.

In another recorded account against a great swordsman who appeared in his finest fighting attire at the agreed-upon time, Musashi purposely showed up late to mentally unfocus his opponent. Musashi was dressed in poor attire. Being late and not following formal protocol of fighting attire unnerved the great swordsman, who Musashi apparently defeated. Musashi again demonstrated using mental advantage to win. He didn't fight using rules or protocol. He fought with principles.

One of the greatest warriors of all time understood the greatest weapon of all was the human mind. This is the same ancient principle noted by Sun Tzu who related thousands of years ago that those who win every battle are not the most skillful. Those who are able to render another army helpless without fighting are the best of all, according to Sun Tzu.

IN THE DOJO

Another black belt and I were teaching class for Master Johnny Miller, who owned the dojo. Master Miller strode onto the mat and began to demonstrate a technique he wanted us to begin drilling the students on that evening.

The technique involved a few strikes then ended with a final strike to the groin. He approached a few students and demonstrated on each of them coming very close to the groin with the final strike. The pupils of their eyes widened but they never moved, as Master Miller stopped short of making contact with each individual demonstration.

He then demonstrated on the last student, who was new to class. When Master Miller stopped his strike just short of this student's groin, the student flinched in fear and stepped back, commenting that the strike had been terribly close.

The other students chuckled a bit and asked the student if he was wearing a protective groin cup. After a quizzical look from the new student, the other students tapped their protective groin cups under their karate uniforms showing they were protected from a strike to the groin if it made contact.

The student looked at Master Miller and asked if he recommended they wear protective cups to class. Master Miller responded, "I don't know. It's your groin."

Whether avoiding conflict, practicing in a dojo, or engaging in direct combat, preparation is the first vital step. In order to win fights, one must prepare, and how one prepares is an individual decision.

PREPARING FOR PEACE

On May 15, 1994, a study was presented at the Annual Meeting of the Safe School's Coalition in Orlando, Florida. The presentation was entitled, "A School/Curricular Intervention Martial Arts Program for At-Risk Students."[23]

Public School 49 in Brooklyn, New York, experienced the same problem as many schools across the nation. The issue was too many inner-city youth with behavioral problems, social dysfunction, and inadequate coping mechanisms resulting in poor academic performance.

The school instituted a martial arts program for at-risk fourth and fifth graders. The class was taught by a professional sensei and was designed to aid students in developing self-control and discipline. Martial arts instructors emphasized traditional training methods revolving around respect, courtesy, and honesty. The curriculum focused on ways to resolve conflict through discipline.

This was after many other methods to control violent behavior had failed, such as instituting rules of no swearing or fighting and rewarding students for conformity. Students selected for participation in the karate class could only remain if their behavior was acceptable. The first goal was simply to minimize aggressive behavior, such as hitting other students.

After the karate class was instituted, these violent behaviors were easily controlled, and the focus shifted to academics. Participating students demonstrated more attentiveness to schoolwork and assignments. A few students dropped out of the class, but most stayed and showed remarkable improvement in their behavior and academic performance.

Interest in gang membership decreased as well. Glasser's 1986 control theory,[24] which is noted in the study, emphasizes that schools do not fulfill a student's need for belonging and power. In fact, the classroom disempowers students through individual conformity rather than cooperative activities. However, the strict discipline of a martial arts program fulfilled these needs of strength and belonging to a group. Students reported that they did not need a gang anymore. The martial arts class improved their self-esteem.

So while martial arts preparation within schools isn't a magic solution for all at-risk youth, it certainly was a great start at one school. Preparation to fight isn't all about fighting as a result of this and other studies. It is about discipline and securing peace through self-control. Being prepared improves self-confidence and has many benefits mutually exclusive to fighting. The wisdom within the principle of preparation that many times one does not have to fight if one is prepared to fight hasn't changed for centuries.

Simply having a plan isn't enough. Preparation is the ability to implement a plan and is vital to winning.

Award-winning speaker and army veteran Alberto Mella says there are three questions to ask in order to prepare to be a warrior in a garden. What conflict will you face? Why are you fighting? What does victory look like?[25] These are reasonable questions in order to prepare for a fight.

Sun Tzu echoed the true essence of this warrior in the garden preparation: "The art of war teaches us to rely not on the likelihood of the enemy's not coming, but on our readiness to receive him."[26]

NOTES

1. Sun Tzu, *The Art of War and Other Classics of Eastern Thought* (New York: Barnes & Noble, 2013).

2. Sven Kraemer, *Inside the Cold War from Marx to Reagan: An Unprecedented Guide to the Roots, History, Strategies and Key Documents of the Cold War* (Washington, DC: University Press of America, 2015), 392.

3. James Barraclough, *MMA Sport Psychology Manual* (2015), chapter 1, http://believeperform.com.

4. Ronda Rousey, *My Fight/Your Fight* (New York: Reagan Arts, 2015), 42–44.

5. Mike Bohn, "Ronda Rousey: What's Next After Second Straight UFC Loss?" *Rolling Stone Magazine,* January 3, 2017, http://rollingstone.com.

6. Jim Rome, "Frank Martin Talks Sweet 16, Duke, and More with Jim Rome," March 21, 2017, *CBS Radio Local,* http://webcache.googleusercontent.com/search?q=cache:itTX4RmY6BkJ:jimrome.com/2017/03/21/frank-martin-talks-sweet-16-duke-and-more-with-jim-rome/+&cd=2&hl=en&ct=clnk&gl=us&client=safari.

7. Sun Tzu, *The Art of War and Other Classics of Eastern Thought* (New York: Barnes & Noble, 2013).

8. Haha Lung, *Mind Control: The Ancient Art of Psychological Warfare* (New York: Kensington Publishing, 2006), 80–82.

9. Robert Nelson, *Inspirational Lessons from Inspirational People* (Morrisville, NC: Lulu Press, 2012).

10. Kent Thune, "Plato—The Philosopher King" (2010), http://financialphilosopher.typepad.com/thefinancialphilosopher/2007/09/plato.html.

11. Barbara Mikkelson, "Inner Golf," *Snopes* (2015), http://www.snopes.com/sports/golf/innergolf.asp.

12. V. K. Ranganathan, V. Siemionow, J. Z. Liu, and G. H. Yue, "From Mental Power to Muscle Power—Gaining Strength by Using the Mind," *Neuropsychologia* 42, no. 7: 944–956.

13. Ibid.

14. Dave Smith, *Disney Trivia from the Vault* (White Plains, New York: Disney Editions, 2012).

15. "One in 100 Children are Psychopaths, Experts Believe," *The Telegraph*, August 31, 2012.

16. Benjamin Gelderen et al., "Psychological Strain and Emotional Labor Among Police-Officers: A Diary Study," *Journal of Vocational Behavior* 71, no. 3 (December 2007): 446–459.

17. Arnold Bakker and Ellen Heuven, "Emotional Dissonance, Burnout, and In-Role Performance Among Nurses and Police Officers," *International Journal of Stress Management* 13 (November 2006): 423–440.

18. Kevin Sites, "The Unforgiven," *Aeon* (2014), https://aeon.co/essays/how-do -soldiers-live-with-their-feelings-of-guilt.

19. Miyamoto Musashi, *The Five Rings, Miyamoto Musashi's Art of Strategy: The New Illustrated Edition of the Japanese Warrior Classic* (New York: Quarto Publishing Group, 2012).

20. "Miyamoto Musashi," *Wikipedia*, last modified June 20, 2017, https://en .wikipedia.org/wiki/Miyamoto_Musashi.

21. Thomas Craig, "The Art of Fighting without Fighting," *Zen Revolution Blog*, January 26, 2013, https://zenrevolution.wordpress.com/2013/01/26/the-art-of -fighting-without-fighting/.

22. "Tsukahara Bokuden," *Wikipedia*, last modified March 26, 2017, https://en .wikipedia.org/wiki/Tsukahara_Bokuden.

23. Jeffrey Glanz, "A School/Curricular Intervention Martial Arts Program for At-Risk Students" (paper presented at the annual meeting of the Safe Schools Coalition, Orlando, Florida, May 15, 1994), https://www.researchgate.net /publication/234682933_A_SchoolCurricular_Intervention_Martial_Arts _Program_for_At-Risk_Students.

24. William Glasser, *Control Theory in the Classroom* (New York: Harper Collins, 1986).

25. Alberto Mella, "The Warrior in the Garden," The Gentlemen's Brotherhood (2017), https://www.thegentlemensbrotherhood.com/inspiration/the-warrior -in-the-garden/.

26. Sun Tzu, *The Art of War*, p. 30.

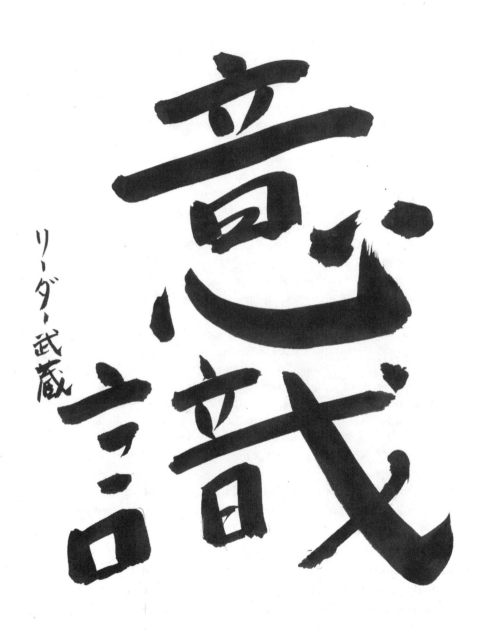

意識

リーダー・武蔵

AWARENESS

AWARENESS IS MORE than simply being alert, though being alert is certainly important. "Alert" is merely seeing. "Awareness" is both seeing and knowing. It is a mind-set in which visual information and clues are processed rather than simply observed.

A deer is alert, but many times will freeze when facing headlights. If the deer possessed an awareness of what caught its attention, the deer wouldn't freeze. The deer would understand to move out of the way. Awareness and alertness must coexist, as the combination is the best self-defense technique to counter the element of surprise. But awareness is the principle that has the deepest cognitive element. Being alert is simply the more rudimentary side of awareness. The overall principle is to try to understand what is being seen in a contextual sense.

The right level of awareness in every situation will hopefully recognize a threat before it has a chance to develop. As noted in Chapter 1, avoiding conflict is the easiest way to win a conflict. This requires the maintenance of a surrounding comfort zone to identify potential threats. These threats can then either be avoided or, if avoidance is impossible, awareness at least provides more time to plan a course of action while robbing the aggressor of the element of surprise. Awareness is the principle that counters surprise and is the first active step after preparation for overcoming conflict.

INATTENTION BLINDNESS

How aware are you? Do you feel like you can multitask well? Do you spot errors in movies? Are you acutely aware of everything going on around you? If you think that you are, then you are probably wrong.

For decades, psychologists have been documenting the many ways perception deceives us. Before experimental psychologists came along, magicians throughout the ages took advantage of perceptual knowledge, utilizing methods like misdirection to easily deceive and amaze.

It seems we can only effectively process a single stream of information at a time. We filter most other information within our awareness out of the picture. This is selective attention or inattentional blindness. Studies have found that the more cognitive effort a task requires, the more likely something will be missed.[1]

The most famous experiment to demonstrate this selective awareness was called "The Invisible Gorilla."[2] Published in 1999 by Christopher Chabris and Daniel Simons, the study involved a video of three people wearing white shirts passing a basketball. There were also three people wearing black shirts passing their own basketball. Participants were asked to count how many times the people in the white shirts passed their ball.

About nine seconds into the video, someone dressed in a gorilla suit walks into the midst of the six people passing the two basketballs, stops, beats his chest, then walks out of the frame on the other side. After the participants watched the video in which they were counting the ball passes, they were asked how many times the ball was passed. They were then asked if they saw anything unusual other than the players. If not, they were then specifically asked if they saw a gorilla. Surprisingly, about half the participants missed seeing the gorilla, though 90 percent of the time people indicated that they would notice something out of the ordinary.

Researchers later utilized an eye tracker to test participants. Those who missed the gorilla actually looked at the gorilla for at least a second. But they still missed it. The psychological literature has recreated this study in different forms many times. The disparity between the richness with which we believe we perceive our experiences and the details we miss is clear.

Looking isn't the same as seeing. Alert isn't the same as aware. Attention must be focused on something to be aware of it. The key is to filter out the distractions that distort our focus of attention. The greater the demand for attention, the less likely we are to notice anything falling outside our focus. During many of the studies on perceptual attention, observers who were not directly engaged in the study with an assigned task upon which to focus clearly saw the gorilla or whatever perceptual item was being tested.

There is no magic answer for countering inattentive blindness. But you can maximize attention by avoiding distractions. You can also make it a habit to notice things others do not. It's not easy and requires practice. You will not notice minute details in the beginning. But you should at least not ignore obvious verbal or visual clues.

PREVENTIVE AWARENESS

Interestingly, the majority of fights come with indications on how to avoid them. A robber who produces a weapon and demands a wallet or someone who instructs his victim to shut up or he'll beat them are both providing instructions on how not to be assaulted. At least in theory, as sometimes the assault comes anyway. There's always the risk. That's why avoidance is 100 percent effective. Once confrontation occurs, anything can happen.

The point is that if given instructions, it isn't wise to make negative comments about the robber's mother. Attention to the information being given is important. Awareness is the tool that helps formulate a plan of action. Awareness allows many opportunities for complete avoidance or deescalation of conflict. If nothing else, awareness buys time.

So being aware is in many ways preventative. It provides time for preparation even if engagement is imminent. It comes with the ability of knowing how to extract yourself from a fight or deny the attacker the element of surprise. Awareness is simply the bridge from preparation to execution of a plan.

Again, most fights come with instructions on how to avoid them. But victims often ignore the instructions as they may not be aware of their options. Ignoring these instructions is usually because of one of the following:

1. Mind-altering substances such as alcohol[3]
2. Ego[4]
3. Stupidity[5]

Eliminating these three variables will eliminate many fights.

To make awareness work, one must know what is going on in the surrounding environment, particularly behind or what may potentially be around the next corner. This is why talking on cell phones, texting, or other preoccupations must be eliminated.

Anything that seems out of place must be noted. Having comprehensive awareness and recognizing things that break normal patterns requires elimination of distractions and constant vigilance. It also requires daily practice.

Being aware of what is going on requires the person to look around a lot.[6] In Vietnam, soldiers were constantly scanning as if their heads were on swivels turning their necks back and forth. It is nearly impossible to close the distance on someone without their knowledge if they have 360-degree awareness. It is not paranoid to always anticipate something happening or monitoring for anything that does not seem right.

While knowing what is around the next corner seems impossible, it can be intuitive. In a bad neighborhood, it is prudent to simply expect something bad around every corner and make a wider berth than would be taken in a crowded mall, for example. In short, give the element of surprise that is typically surrendered to an attacker less opportunity to enter the equation.

TRAGEDY

I served on a rescue team with a young man who had suffered a lethal gunshot wound near a populated mall one night. He had pulled up to a nearby drive-in bank. While making a transaction a thug commissioned with a gang initiation walked up beside his vehicle, shot him, and ran. His vehicle rolled forward into a nearby curb.

I asked a police officer friend about the victim's weapon. The officer was a mutual friend and we both knew that the victim always kept a small handgun tucked in the overhead visor of his vehicle. The officer said as his vehicle bumped into the curb, his weapon fell out of the overhead visor and landed in his lap. He never had time to access it, even though it was so close.

Did the thug hide effectively enough and not give him enough time to react? The ambush clearly happened so quickly that our friend had no time to even think about accessing his nearby weapon. The element of surprise is a powerful thing and it favors the attacker.

Many experts, such as retired police instructor and CIA officer Ed Lovette, would advise that the best reaction in such a situation is to escape.[7] A vehicle weighing over a ton with a large engine is a powerful thing. Stepping on the gas to speed away from an attacker on foot is much quicker than accessing a weapon. But it takes a few seconds to analyze a situation and execute this action.

Massad Ayoob is a preeminent firearms expert who has authored numerous books and more than a thousand articles on firearm techniques. He discusses the same concept in his classic book on the role of the firearms for personal protection, *In the Gravest Extreme*.[8] Even with a weapon in hand, Ayoob recommends always taking advantage of available cover.

The U.S. Marines have a saying that if you're not shooting you should be moving. It's called getting off the X, and is a common military concept. Former CIA protective agent Scott Richardson wrote an entire book on this concept, entitled *Get Off the X: A CIA Agent's Guide to Protecting You and Your Family*.[9] The point is that if awareness alerts you to an imminent threat, the best reaction may be to simply move or escape before engaging in a fight.

Could more awareness have bought my friend more time to react? We will never know. But it is clear that awareness is more important than having a weapon, skill, or nearly any other principle or defense tool. Awareness must be implemented before any tool can be deployed effectively. Awareness may be the principle that determines if other principles can be executed at all.

AWARENESS OF A SPY

Being aware doesn't necessarily mean being paranoid. It simply means not being otherwise preoccupied or self-absorbed. The preoccupation should be with surroundings, by scanning and becoming interested in the environment.

There is a brilliant scene demonstrating a supreme level of awareness by screenwriter Tony Gilroy in the movie *The Bourne Identity*.[10] The hero, played by Matt Damon, reveals how acutely aware he is of his surroundings. He is trying to understand what type of training he had in the past. He confesses that even though he is sitting in a peaceful restaurant, he habitually has developed a sense of knowing how many people are in the establishment, which ones might be a potential threat, which ones may be armed, how many vehicles are out front, and how quickly he can make a hasty exit if necessary. He isn't paranoid. He simply catalogs this information unconsciously and habitually.

You already know how to be aware. The U.S. Secret Service doesn't just teach how to identify a counterfeit bill. They also teach what a normal bill should look like as a comparison.

Knowing what is normal is easier than fathoming the thousands of other options. The same method applies to what everyone already knows about his or her surroundings.

You already know what is normal around you. If a strange face arrives at your door or an odd package is left alone it should arouse suspicion as it breaks the normal pattern. But some things are so subtle that only a keen sense of awareness will note them.

A car that matches your speed as you drive is subtle but suspicious. Someone who seems to move once they spot you is subtle but suspicious. Any actions of this type must be explained or be prepared for countermeasures.

A common ploy used by predators is to gain the confidence of a victim. They may match the movements of the victim, stalk them slowly, and ask for directions or a cigarette in an attempt to get closer and closer. Their conversation is designed cleverly to lower the victim's awareness or suspicion. They know the magician's skill of misdirection. The predator may even be polite at first. Many predators will not exhibit threatening behavior until it is too late. Their calm mannerisms are intended to break through outer regions of personal space.

THE ZONE

Varying levels of awareness must surround this personal comfort zone. Being wary of anyone trying to penetrate this zone is only practical. The closer someone gets, the more suspicious you should become. Never let anyone get too close. Question all credentials or information a person provides in an attempt to penetrate a personal zone. Never go around a corner or open a door you can't fully see beyond, both literally and figuratively.

Bruce Lee recognized that being aware of one's surroundings was far from being paranoid. He called it, "being wholly and quietly alive . . . aware and alert, ready for whatever may come."[11] This type of awareness allows a greater appreciation for our immediate surroundings.

FRIEND OR FOE

Awareness specifically allows discernment of threats, which means identifying what will harm and what will not harm. This is the information that should constantly be filtered.

This friend-versus-foe philosophy is not only a natural inclination, but an ancient truth. Luke 11:23 recorded the observation that he who isn't with me is against me. Aristotle recognized the necessity of assessing character to distinguish friend from foe.[12] Even the infamous German political theorist Carl Schmitt noted that the high point of politics was the moment that the enemy in all its clarity was recognized as the enemy.[13] The intention to help or harm differentiates friend from foe. Sometimes it can be difficult telling the good guys from the bad guys. Everyone who tries to help may not be your friend. Everyone who seems to hurt may not be your enemy.

This truth has been written about for centuries. But every fighter should strive to identify the enemy. This may seem obvious, but many times it is not immediately evident.

"Keep your friends close and your enemies closer" is a classic quote from the Francis Ford Coppola film *The Godfather*. It is important to know your enemy before he realizes that you know he is an enemy. Keeping them close was the godfather's way of being more aware of what his enemies were doing.

A clear distinction between friend and foe is a fundamental concept to winning fights. Gray areas in between are often accepted in politics and social situations. The concept is a bit different in nonphysical self-defense, as in politics where keeping your friends close and your enemies closer has varying degrees of value depending on whether they are identified and revealed as an enemy. Keeping enemies close for information has a tactical advantage as ambiguity can be helpful in these situations.

But with strangers or physical confrontations, the distinction between friend and foe must be swift and clear. There must be no ambiguity. An enemy must be identified as such, and action must be swift. Awareness makes this distinction. It's all about situational context.

During the heat of battle the mind tends to lose its balance. Differentiating friend from foe provides not only distance from enemies but focus for the fighter's own mind. No quarter can be given to an enemy seeking to harm. Trying to justify that an enemy may be a friend, and the hesitation this may cause, could be costly. Enemies can generally be quickly identified by their actions. Friends take longer to prove good intent. Unfortunately, the reality is that a track record must develop before a fighter can let his guard down. But even then a fighter must remain alert and aware. Awareness involves a healthy dose of skepticism.

The local sheriff is a good friend. I remember when he was a rookie cop. I worked in the communications division as a dispatcher of the same police department while working my way through college. He related a story to me once about a local man we both knew who had Asperger's syndrome. His name was Ed. Ed rode a bike around town equipped with a citizens band radio. He wore a green military jacket with an outback-style hat stained with sweat and smoked a pipe. In the early 1980s he also slung a shotgun over his shoulder.

The local police knew him well, as he was a friend of local law enforcement. He wasn't a local threat to anyone. He'd stop by the police department to clean their guns and generally hang out with those of us working the night shift in the communications division.

The sheriff recalled stopping two individuals in a vehicle one night as a rookie officer. He got the driver out of the vehicle and was conducting a sobriety test in the front of the vehicle leaving the passenger inside.

Suddenly, he heard Ed's voice. "Mister, don't make that fatal mistake."

Looking toward the back of the vehicle just behind the passenger door he saw Ed in his stained hat, pipe clenched between his teeth, with his shotgun shouldered. It appeared at first glance that Ed was pointing the shotgun at the officer.

The future sheriff paused only because he knew Ed wasn't a threat. Ed would never point a gun at an officer. He then heard the passenger door slam.

Ed had quietly ridden his bike up to the traffic stop. No one saw Ed in the darkness. Ed then saw the passenger slowly open his door and start to quietly exit as the sobriety test was being given to the driver a few feet away. It was then that Ed made his way to the rear of the vehicle unseen, shouldered his shotgun, and announced his warning to the passenger from the right rear of the vehicle.

Realizing Ed was pointing the weapon at the passenger between them, the officer also drew his weapon on the passenger and ordered him out of the vehicle. It was then that a weapon was found under the passenger seat where the passenger had tossed it upon slamming the door shut.

The sheriff says Ed saved his life that night. The sheriff had known Ed so long that this friendship had established Ed was not a threat to him as again, a friend's intention takes longer to establish than an enemy's. Ed's life was also saved. Another officer may have determined Ed was a threat in the fraction of a second when an officer must make a decision.

In the heat of the moment, it is often difficult to differentiate friend from foe. It can sometimes be a complex exercise. But understanding who poses a real threat is important.

INTERNAL AWARENESS

Much of this ability requires internal awareness as well. Emotions can be much more intense than rationality. Self-discipline is necessary to maintain a presence of mind capable of awareness that allows us to focus our emotions and make rational decisions.

Notice the concept isn't to control or suppress emotion as much as to focus it. This subtle concept will be of greater importance regarding other principles that require channeling of emotion for precise effect. It is noted here only to understand that discerning friend from foe must sometimes be more a logical task than an emotional one. It also is an acknowledgment that emotional responses are inevitable. Self-discipline prevents emotions from becoming overwhelming. Focusing on awareness or a single task prevents feelings of panic to take root. Also, if you can force your opponent to be more emotional than you, the foe will be unbalanced.

Self-awareness requires much discipline until it becomes habit. A fighter must have complete self-control to have complete control of his environmental awareness. Self-awareness is a vital skill. Sun Tzu said, "If you know the enemy and know yourself, you need not fear the result of a hundred battles."[14]

CONFLICT RESOLUTION

Fighters must be aware that there are only about six logical ways to resolve conflict. These six ways of dealing with conflict have been modeled extensively in various disciplines and by many models with a universal approach in the context of friend or foe awareness.[15] The following are ways to resolve conflict according to a consensus of these models:

1. **Avoidance or otherwise escape.** Resolution is not achieved but the immediate danger is avoided. In business, this is a lose-lose situation but in a physical environment this is a win for the intended victim.
2. **Fight to win.** This method is about overwhelming and conquering an enemy or opponent. Someone has to win and someone has to lose. The option doesn't necessarily appear in all models but is the clear objective in a fight.
3. **Concede or retreat.** Giving up one's position admits defeat and automatically loses. It is a lose-win situation.
4. **Evasion of responsibility or delegation.** Delegating responsibility to someone else is a common method of dealing with conflict. Usually, this delegation is to a higher authority that resolves the conflict on behalf of the parties. The danger is that the conflict may not be resolved in the best interest of either party.
5. **Compromise.** Arriving at a solution that is acceptable to both parties is sometimes not ideal, but can be a reasonable method.

6. **Consensus.** This contrasts with a compromise in that a new solution is achieved and no one has to concede anything. Both parties have agreed on a different solution. This is a win-win situation.

Do not confuse the above principles of conflict resolution as being applicable to all violent confrontations. If the situation has risen to the level of violence it may be too late for most of these methods, as the options are narrowed to either escape or fight to win. An understanding of all the models of conflict resolution is necessary before escape or violence is the only viable option.

IN THE DOJO

Dr. James West is a medical doctor and attorney who is also a fellow black belt. One evening, he and I were teaching a martial arts class for Master Johnny Miller.

A new student arrived who was interested in trying our class. He was a big guy and said he was a department of corrections officer. Toward the end of class West and I split the class up for a bit of sparring. We were trying to figure out who to let spar with whom when the new student pointed at a small girl in the corner whom we'll call Casey. She was a green belt and had been with us for years. "Can I spar with the little lady?" he asked. He then grinned and chuckled a bit.

I looked past West and over at Master Miller. We usually only let black belts spar with new students. It was a class rule. Black belts can control their actions and wouldn't hurt a new member of class. Master Miller and I had both studied with Master Nathaniel Thompson. This was one of his rules. He warned that if you beat up on your students, they won't come back to play with you.

Master Miller was leaning on a punching bag. He rubbed his gray hair and nodded. I looked at the new guy and told him that would be okay.

"I was just joking. I don't want to hurt the little girl," he said.

I explained she knew how to handle herself. It would be fine. They lined up and we let them begin. Casey dodged in, landed blows, and quickly retreated beyond the new guy's lumbering reach. He was never able to lay a glove on her. She did this relentlessly.

I could tell he was getting frustrated and asked if he was okay.

"Well, I'm a corrections officer. I'm trained to subdue prisoners, not spar with them. That's what I'm good at," he said.

I looked over at Master Miller. Should we let him grapple on his first night with Casey? Master Miller smiled. He then nodded.

The new guy was then instructed that if he could get his hands on Casey and if he could take her down, they could grapple at that point. The guy switched from trying to hit Casey to trying to grab her. Casey eluded his grasp for a while until suddenly he grabbed the fabric of her karate gi.

Casey tugged but he held on. He was much stronger than she was and when he tugged back it nearly lifted Casey off her feet. As he tugged Casey toward him, Casey not only went along with his pull, but suddenly spun her back to him while holding his arm. She then reached her other arm under his armpit. Everyone knew what was coming except the new guy as she quickly shifted her hip into him while pulling his arm and bending over slightly. It was the most beautiful hip throw I think I've ever seen. Her hip became a fulcrum.

One second the guy's feet were firmly planted on the ground pulling on a girl a fraction of his size. The next second he was airborne, legs flailing through the air.

He bounced as he hit the mat. But Casey wasn't finished. As he was still trying to figure out what happened, Casey pressed his arm to her chest. She threw her legs on either side of his arm, crossing them across his chest at the ankles, then dropped onto her back pulling his arm with all her might. His arm straightened. She pulled hard while lying on her back clutching his arm and lifting her hips against his elbow.

I leaned over them. His face was red. He was straining to get his arm back to no avail. It was then that I realized we might not have oriented him to the grappling rules yet.

I explained, "Sir. If you tap that little girl's leg three times she will let you go. Otherwise, I think she's going to break your arm."

He tapped. She let go. He never came back to class.

There are a couple of points besides the fact that this is a funny story. First, Master Thompson was right. You should never beat up on a new student or they won't come back. But the most important is that not only must a fighter be aware of the surroundings. A fighter must also be aware of his or her own capabilities. It goes back to internal awareness.

Your training, capabilities, and whether escape is an option determine if you can run or must fight. Being aware of threats and options to handle those threats is essential.

Our new student arrived with preconceived notions of his own capabilities. He wasn't aware of his own limitations. He certainly wasn't aware of the capabilities of other students half his size with much more training. The point is to take nothing for granted when it comes to awareness. Be externally and internally aware. Be wary of everything including little girls named Casey wearing green belts.

How do you acquire Jason Bourne level awareness? You practice.

PRACTICE AWARENESS

Putting these things together means incorporating awareness into daily activities. Identifying dangers takes a lot of practice. You aren't looking for trouble; you are looking for ways to avoid it. Here's a system to consider:

1. Assess
   a. Note surroundings and evaluate every situation you find yourself in. Identify risks; escape routes, dangers, and distractions.
   b. Understand the potential threat level of each identified risk.
   c. Make sure you are looking around in a 360-degree arc.
2. Establish a Baseline
   a. Know what is normal in the environment that surrounds you. Someone in an overcoat on a sunny day would be out of place. Situations, behaviors, sights and sounds that are out of place should be noted.
3. Plan
   a. Mentally prepare yourself for dangerous situations. If a group of people seems to cross the street and walk toward you, how will you escape? Decide before the potential threat is close. Decide what you will do when it is observed and still a potential threat.
4. Eliminate Distractions
   a. Texting and talking on a phone prevents 360-degree awareness.

b. Fully experience your surroundings distraction-free. Note not only sights and sounds but also smells or things that don't feel right. Distractions prevent utilization of all your senses on the surroundings as a whole.

5. Time and Space Awareness
   a. Be conscious of how long it has been since you saw companions you may be accompanying. Are they late? Why has that person been standing across the road watching you for so long? Does this person mirror your movements and walk when you walk? Know where you are at all times and where you can potentially move to if needed. Know how long it will take this to happen.
   b. Use peripheral vision, mirrors, and windows to casually scan surroundings.
   c. Do you know where the exits are located? Do you know where to find weapons? Is the space friendly or hostile?

6. Focus
   a. Don't become mentally fatigued, allowing the mind to wander. Never get too complacent in comfortable surroundings.

7. Positioning
   a. Remember the old Western movies where the cowboy always wanted his back to the wall so he could watch the door? There's a lot of wisdom in that method. Being able to watch people as they approach or positioning near exits for a quick escape especially in a crowded environment is wise.

8. Maintain a Safe Zone
   a. No one should be allowed within a few feet of your personal space. If they do, then they must be identified as friend or foe quickly. Any threat they may pose must be determined. Look for signs of a weapon and where they are looking. Watch their hands. Hands and eyes will reveal their intent.

Most awareness methods have similar themes. Eliminating distractions and focusing on surroundings looking for what doesn't fit is key. Then make sure you are in a position to either fight or escape. There are other approaches that demonstrate awareness in action but you get the idea. Eliminating distractions and gaining as much information about your surroundings is vital. With practice, it is not only fun but will also soon become instinctive.

AWARENESS METHODOLOGY

Observe, Orient, Decide, Act is the OODA loop system developed by military strategist and U.S. Air Force fighter pilot John Boyd.[16] The person who can cycle through this loop the quickest typically wins.

Observe and Orient is the awareness part of this cycle. Observing is taking in the surroundings. Orienting is noting what we are observing in context. We first must orient in context to know what to do with the observations. We will discuss the rest of the OODA loop a bit later. For now, understand that half this loop involves awareness.

There are various methods of threat awareness. Some are color coded. Others are numbered. There are levels that call for being relaxed yet alert as there is no specific threat. Then it escalates as the threats become imminent. They are all good labeling methods.

The magic of any model is to simply maintain an awareness that coincides with the threat potential. The higher the potential, the higher the awareness, though awareness should never drop to zero.

In *Left of Bang: How the Marine Corps' Combat Hunter Program Can Save Your Life*, Patrick Van Horne describes domains of human behavior that are used on the battlefield to quickly determine friend or foe status of a potential threat.[17] It is a good model for awareness methodology. Though we've alluded to noting anomalies in general, there are three main body language groups that help provide a basis for anomalies in particular as described by Horne:

1. Dominant / Submissive Behavior
   a. Most people try to be friendly for the most part. Anyone trying to assert dominance should therefore be considered an anomaly of the normal environment and a potential threat. We've already discussed how this breaks normal patterns.
2. Comfortable / Uncomfortable Behavior
   a. Most people are relaxed in most situations. People who are threats may tend to look nervous or look around to see if anyone

is looking at them. This is an anomaly and a potential threat. Also note anyone who is calm when everyone else is not. The Boston Marathon bombers were easily identified on film, as they were calm while everyone else was running in a panic.

    b. Police will check the hands of suspicious persons who seem to want to reach for something nervously. Hands and eyes often reveal if a person is accessing a weapon or about to strike.

3. Interested / Uninterested Behavior

    a. Most people aren't paying attention to things around them. Anyone showing specific interest in a person or object is an anomaly and should be noted.

PLAN AWARENESS

Once an anomaly is spotted, have a plan. This involves utilizing the information gathered while being aware. If someone enters a restaurant with a gun while you are having lunch, then you should know where the nearest exit is located. Hopefully, you have positioned yourself near the exit so you can watch the area. Remember, if you decide to take out a threat by whatever means, when the police arrive they must identify whether or not you are a threat as well. Anyone holding a gun, knife, or standing over a bloody body will be understandably suspicious until they sort out the good guys from the bad guys.

PLAN EXECUTION

If you are a fighter and have watched fight films of your opponent, you know every time he delivers a front kick he drops his hands. You may plan to counter the first time you see a front kick. In a crowded restaurant, you may sit down with a plan to dash out the back door if trouble starts at the front.

Whatever the situation that may lead to a potential or planned fight, being aware garners information that can be used to formulate a plan. Awareness requires practice for this to become a habit. Awareness will trigger your plan.

There is no magic formula. There is no perfect method. There is no fool-proof way to completely combat the element of surprise, which is the enemy of awareness. But eliminating distractions and practicing Jason Bourne level awareness soon becomes a habit that minimizes threats.

NOTES

1. Duncan E. Astle and Gaia Scerif, "Using Developmental Cognitive Neuroscience to Study Behavioral and Attentional Control," *Developmental Psychology*, no. 51 (March 2009): 107–118.

2. Daniel Simons and Christopher Chabris, "Gorillas in Our Midst: Sustained Inattentional Blindness for Dynamic Events," *Perception* 28, no. 9 (1999): 1059–1074.

3. Bruchas et al., "Selective P38a MAPK Deletion in Serotonergic Neurons Produces Resilience in Models of Depression and Addiction," *Neuron*, no. 71 (August 2011): 498–511.

4. Roy Baumeister, Laura Smart, and Joseph Boden, "Relation of Threatened Egotism to Violence and Aggression: The Dark Side of High Self Esteem," *Psychological Review*, no. 1 (January 1996): 5–33.

5. Aczel Balazs, Palfi Bence, and Zoltan Kekecs, "What Is Stupid?: People's Conception of Unintelligent Behavior," *Intelligence*, no. 53 (2015): 51–58.

6. United States Marine Corps Manual, *Scouting and Patrolling Operations* (Quantico, VA: The Basic School Marine Corps Training Command), http://www.trngcmd.marines.mil/Portals/207/Docs/TBS/W2D0001XQ-DM%20Scouting%20and%20Patrolling%20Operations.pdf?ver=2016-01-26-112649-563.

7. Ed Lovette, "Surviving Vehicle Ambushes," *Police: The Law Enforcement Magazine*, October 17, 2011, http://www.policemag.com/channel/vehicles/articles/2011/10/surviving-vehicle-ambushes.aspx.

8. Massad Ayoob, *In the Gravest Extreme* (Concord, NH: Police Bookshelf, 1980).

9. Scott Richardson, *Get Off the X: A CIA Agent's Guide to Protecting You and Your Family* (Morrisville, NC: Lulu Press Online, 2016).

10. Doug Liman, dir., *The Bourne Identity*. Screenplay by Tony Gilroy. Based on a book by Robert Ludlum (2002), http://www.dailyscript.com/scripts/bourne identity.html.

11. Bruce Lee, *The Tao of Jeet Kune Do* (Santa Clarita, CA: Ohara, 1975).

12. Graeme Watson, Barbara Renzi, Elisabetta Viggiani, and Mairead Collins, *Friends and Foes Volume 1: Friendship and Conflict in Philosophy and the Arts* (Newcastle upon Tyne, UK: Cambridge Scholars Publishing, 2009), 24.

13. "Carl Schmitt," Wikiquote, last modified March 31, 2017, https://en.wiki quote.org/wiki/Carl_Schmitt, and Robert Greene, *The 33 Strategies of War* (New York: Penguin, 2006).
14. Sun Tzu, *The Art of War and Other Classics of Eastern Thought* (New York: Barnes & Noble, 2013).
15. C-T. Bayer and B. T. Schernick, "Conflict Management Module," *Friedrich Ebert Stiftung Youth Leadership Development Programme*, http://library.fes .de/pdf-files/bueros/namibia/05912.pdf.
16. "OODA Loop," Wikipedia, last modified June 9, 2017, https://en.wikipedia .org/wiki/OODA_loop.
17. Patrick Van Horne and Jason A. Riley, *Left of Bang* (New York: Black Irish Entertainment, 2014).

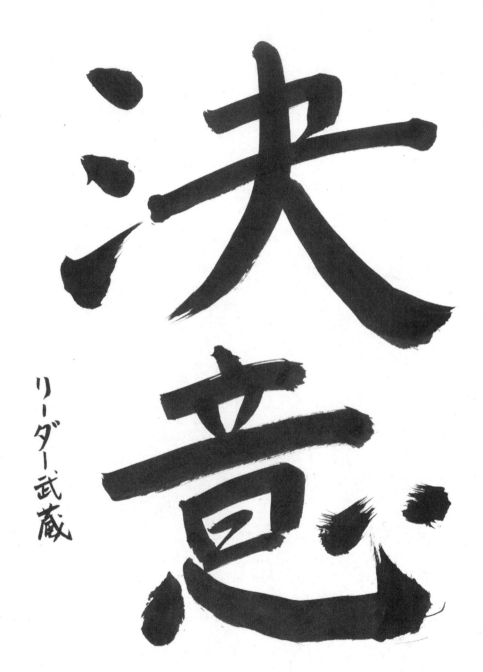

決意

リーダー武蔵

COMMITMENT

THE PRINCIPLES OF preparation and awareness provide the fighter with the opportunity to avoid a fight or deny the opponent the opportunity of surprise if avoidance is not an option. But at some point, a decision must be reached regarding action. The fighter must then be fully committed to this action to be successful.

In the short term this is being decisive. It is focused determination. There must be complete commitment to the decision once action is necessary. The full depth of commitment cannot be emphasized enough as it applies to this principle. It is making an unwavering decision then focusing on a course of action with vigor. Commitment is a sense of seeing the task to fruition regardless of the obstacles encountered. Martial artists recognize the concept as striking through the target and committing to breaking it.

Striking through a target means you are still accelerating when you reach the target. The fighter stops accelerating only when the goal has been achieved. A committed runner does the same thing. A runner committed to winning a race does not slow down as he is reaching the finish line. He runs through the finish line as hard as he can because he is committed until the end.

It is a combination of striking an object (decisive) and striking through an object (commitment). To break a board you certainly must be decisive.

But more important, you also must be committed. Every martial artist understands the power that is achieved with follow through. It is fine to decide to strike, but striking through the objective results in true commitment and power. This is the interplay of decisiveness and commitment.

SUN TZU

There is a story regarding Sun Tzu who was challenged by the King of Wu to put Sun Tzu's theory of managing soldiers to the test. The king asked if his principles could be applied to women, which was unheard of at the time.

Sun Tzu agreed and was given 180 women from the palace to train. He divided them into two companies and placed the king's favorite concubines at the head of each group. They then were told to follow instructions in unison to begin marching drills.

But when he ordered them to turn left or to turn right the women simply laughed, refusing to obey the orders. They agreed that they understood the instructions but nevertheless they simply giggled. Sun Tzu said that if the words were not clear and distinct or if the orders were not clearly understood, then the general was to blame. But since the orders are clear, the soldiers admit they understand them yet disobey, then it is the fault of their officers.[1]

Sun Tzu ordered the women who led each group to be beheaded. When the king learned his two favorite concubines were about to be executed he tried to intervene. Sun Tzu would not let the king stop the executions. He advised the king that upon accepting his majesty's commission to be general of his forces, there were certain commands from the king he could not accept in order to fulfill his commitment to the king. The two concubines were executed.

Sun Tzu then installed two new leaders. Both groups then drilled in perfect precision. Sun Tzu sent a messenger to inform the king that his troops were now properly disciplined and ready for inspection. He said the troops were ready to obey any order and would walk through fire or water if required by the king. But that isn't the end to the lesson of Sun Tzu.

The king sent word back that Sun Tzu could cease drilling and return to his camp and that he had no need to inspect Sun Tzu's work with the troops. Whereupon Sun Tzu said that the king was only fond of words and could not translate them into deeds. Ultimately, the King of Wu appointed Sun Tzu as his general. They then defeated the surrounding providences under his leadership.

Sun Tzu was a man of action. Objectives were focused and serious to him. He was clearly decisive in his actions and committed to a choice of action once decided upon.

It is interesting to note that the philosophy at the time of Sun Tzu wasn't simply warlike. A document that survived from the Han period and included in the short preface of Ts'ao's edition of Sun Tzu's *Art of War* noted that a ruler who relies solely on warlike measures will be exterminated. But one who relies solely on peaceful measures shall perish as well.[2] Force is used when driven by necessity, but must be used when the occasion requires it. This balance must be understood in the context of committing to action whether in peace or war.

KARATE KID

Lessons of commitment are demonstrated in many iconic films. In the movie *The Karate Kid*, screenwriter Robert Mark Kamen crafted a scene in which Mr. Miyagi provided a glimpse into the type of commitment necessary to win fights and the serious implications of not fully committing to action. He says to his student, "Either you karate do 'yes' or karate do 'no.' You karate do 'guess so . . .'" he then makes a squishing gesture. Mr. Miyagi adds that walking on the left side of the road is fine and walking on the right side is fine. But if you don't pick a side and walk down the middle you soon will be squashed. The fighter must have this decisive commitment. Choosing the middle of the road or doing things halfway will fail. But even more than total commitment, the action must be swift and vigorously executed with firm resolve. This is the decisive element of commitment.

COMMIT FULLY

According to General George S. Patton, "A good plan violently executed now is better than a perfect plan executed next week."[3] The concept is similar to an old marine adage that it is necessary to be aggressive enough, quickly enough. Both the character of Mr. Miyagi and General Patton illustrated the dangers of indecision. Even if the decision isn't perfect, indecision can be worse. Committing fully to the decided action is vital for success.

Action on a decision must be executed without hesitation. Sometimes it isn't what you do as much as how forcefully you do it that makes the action successful. This requires purposeful determination with the intent to end conflict swiftly.

Being committed to a course of action means not wavering in that decision. The decision in the matter is over and all force must be brought to bear on a course of action along with a proper follow through. In other words, commitment to an action must not only connect. It must be so decisive it pierces through the target, as the aim is to be intense and purposeful.

IN THE DOJO

A fighter is trained not to simply hit an object but to commit so fully to the action that he strikes through it. As an under belt, I recall entering our dojo training hall to see a small solid cinderblock resting between two larger ones. My instructor was Master Miller, and he casually indicated that I was to break the block before class began. I had broken a few boards in training, but never a cinder block. I had seen it done though.

I lined up, took a few breaths and practice strikes, then focusing on the block struck it hard with my fist the way I had been trained, or so I thought. My hand hit with a thud. It hurt. My hand fortunately didn't break but neither did the cinderblock.

"What did you do wrong?" Master Miller said.

"I didn't strike through it," I said.

He nodded and said that I must not aim at the cinder block but through it. I should strike through it purposefully and commit fully to the action without hesitation or doubt. By simply striking at it, I'm not fully committed or certain in my mind that it will break. Commitment begins with committed thoughts followed by decisive action. A fighter must fully commit to the decision with certainty that it will succeed.

By striking through it, I'm committing to a decisive action that will break it. There is a huge difference between striking a target and striking through a target. The next time I struck the block, I aimed through it, not at it. It broke. It also was painless.

The point is that uncertainty vanishes when you are committed to an action. You must be mentally certain you will succeed. This provides the focus needed to accomplish the task. But again, decisive action must be swift. Hesitation is not an option in a fight. This applies to the broader concept of a fighter training for a fight that requires months of commitment to prepare. It applies to the fight itself, when every blow must be a decisive commitment.

MENTALLY BURN THE SHIPS

In 1519, upon landing in Veracruz to begin a great conquest, Captain Hernan Cortez ordered his men to burn the ships.[4] Without the ships they had no way home. They had no other option but to succeed in the new world they were about to conquer.

Captain Cortez understood the value of total commitment. Retreat is easy if that is an option. But in Cortez's view, failure was not an option. The expedition would either succeed or fail with no ships available to return home. There was no middle ground. His conquest was the start of the Spanish Empire, which lasted 400 years. The action solidified his troops' commitment to success.

Practicing this principle can be difficult, and we can be our own worst enemies due to our natural tendency to hesitate or take the easy way out. Commitment can be difficult as we are always filled with doubt. Captain Cortez understood his troops would have doubts about winning in a foreign land against all odds. Maybe they would sometimes be outnumbered. Would they fight if a greater force met them? Cortez removed all doubt. His men would either win or perish. This created resolve and incredible commitment.

Many of us worry about the future. We hesitate. The winning strategy is to forcefully engage the present, which will often take care of the future. If a fighter hesitates because he is uncertain about the future outcome of an action, then he is not fully engaged in the present. Like Cortez, fighters must burn all the options that prevent this type of thinking because it only wastes time and resources.

Corrie ten Boom was a Christian and Dutch watchmaker who helped Jews escape the Holocaust during World War II and was imprisoned for her actions. She once said, "Worrying is carrying tomorrow's load with today's strength—carrying two days at once. It is moving into tomorrow ahead of time. Worrying doesn't empty tomorrow of its sorrow, it empties today of its strength."[5] Corrie ten Boom knew a lot about committing focus.

The Hagakure is a collection of commentaries written by Samurai Yamamoto Tsunetomo between 1709 and 1716. In one passage he relates the view of Lord Naoshige, who said, "The way of the Samurai is in desperateness. Ten men or more cannot kill such a man."[6] He further notes this mind-set as simply becoming insane and desperate. It is a much misunderstood warrior code.

The Samurai resolved that they were willing to die at any moment. It is this willingness to sacrifice that Naoshige referred to as desperation. He doesn't use it in the context of surrender. He uses the term "desperation" in the context of the whole world being against you, or a cornered animal that becomes mad, insane, and incredibly violent. The animal cannot easily be defeated due to its commitment to win the fight that emerges from desperation. It is desperation to win, because there is no other option.

Practicing with desperation provides alertness and commitment to action when presented with an insurmountable situation. Desperation will cause a fighter to do things he otherwise would not do. Desperation is an explosive need for action in the face of despair. The Samurai understood this odd emotion. Few fighters today attempt to understand or access desperation, which can provide the single-minded focus of commitment they need. Certainly, Cortez's men began fighting with desperation knowing they had no method of escape. Fighting with desperation is a powerful thing. It is a special kind of commitment to action that makes a fighter unstoppable if he is able to tap into it like the Samurai.

Soldiers who have engaged in close quarters combat during wartime understand this concept. It is in desperation that they fight or die. It is also this desperate mind-set that drives a soldier to perform incredible feats of violence that he might otherwise think he is incapable of performing. But in desperation one will do anything to survive. It is this desperate mind-set, the commitment to win at all costs, that the Samurai purposefully sought when entering battle.

There is another concept found in the Hagakure regarding accepting the present and acting accordingly without wasting resources. It involves the paradoxical inner calmness and focus that must accompany fighting with desperation.

Tsunetomo touches on this concept, relating that there is something that can be learned from a rainstorm. He describes in detail how we try not to get wet by running or passing under the eaves of houses. But we still get wet. He relates that the Samurai must be resolved from the beginning that he will get wet. Then even if he becomes soaked in a rainstorm, the Samurai will not be perplexed or worried about it. This is the understanding that futile efforts will not change the outcome and will only make it worse. It isn't about giving up. It is the opposite. It parallels the concept of desperation. It is about ensuring there is no wasted motion and accepting that the rain isn't all that bad. It is about resolve and doing what must be done despite the circumstances. It's Corrie ten Boom not worrying about tomorrow. To the Samurai, not worrying about the rain is an excellent visual analogy. Accepting today and committing to action now despite the difficulty and regardless of tomorrow also creates inner peace for warriors who engage in violent action.

Despite the rain, we should focus on committing to our goal and not worry about the little things that may get in the way of that goal. This is focused commitment. It is resolve. It is a resolve that enables the Samurai to walk calmly in the rain and not worry about getting wet. He has decided that getting wet is simply part of being in a rainstorm.

The Samurai also accepted they might die in battle. You see it as a recurring theme in literature surrounding the Samurai. They speak of welcoming death. It was a part of life. Death was not an enemy to the Samurai who were not fatalistic. They did not fear death on the battlefield. They simply possessed an inner peace regarding death.

It wasn't courage either. It was commitment to the task or battle at hand and an acceptance of any possibility that may come. Death was then nothing to worry about or fear. It is the same mental calmness just as they accepted that if it rained they would get wet walking in a storm with their head held in the same manner as if it were sunny. Death and rain were simply characters and both ceased to be an enemy with this thinking. Neither one bothered the Samurai. Why should they be bothered if both were inevitable?

This is reminiscent of MMA Fighter Ronda Rousey, who believes pain is just information. To the Samurai, whether it is death or rain it is simply something to accept but not something that will alter the decided course of action when one is completely committed to the task.

Paradoxically, it was difficult to kill a Samurai due to this resolve. Neither death nor rain mattered, and when you remove what doesn't matter, the mind is clear to focus and commit to the goal that is really important. When you think about the power of that attitude, it is difficult to stop anyone who possesses it.

PHYSICS

The physical aspect of commitment is clear. Isaac Newton's second law of motion dictates that acceleration multiplied by mass equals force (ma = F).[7] The math is pretty simple. It explains how a small guy like Bruce Lee, who was 5 foot 7 and weighed 141 pounds, could hit harder than a massive guy. If you double acceleration you increase force in the same ratio as if you doubled mass.

If you are striking a target decisively with committed action then you are striking through the target. If you are striking through the target then you are still accelerating any mass you are putting behind the strike when it reaches its target. If you are striking at the target rather than through the target you lose part of this acceleration, which is multiplied by mass to create the force. Using your whole body and striking through a target optimizes force.

More about speed later. But committing to action certainly helps mathematically by continuing to accelerate force through the target.

WARRIOR COMMITMENT

Miyamoto Musashi specifically said a warrior must be decisive.[8] He urged warriors to train constantly in order to make quick decisions.

There is a Latin proverb that says, "Deliberate often—Decide once."[9] By training constantly, you know your capabilities. By understanding the proper warrior mind-set, you know your values. Knowledge of your physical and mental capabilities can help direct your action by deliberating what you should or should not do in a given situation.

It has been emphasized often that a fighter learns to fight so he doesn't have to fight. It is an old paradox. As a warrior, words are not wasted and actions are not frivolous. A warrior is measured. He deliberates. Then his actions are decisive according to his ability, values, and intent.

There is a lot of emphasis in the ancient literature regarding the seemingly morbid fixation of the Samurai on their approach to death. But it only seems morbid in Western thought. The Eastern attitude is like that of a Samurai walking in the rain not caring about the water, or Ronda Rousey opining that pain is only information. The attitude of the Samurai toward death is that it simply is a reminder to seize the moment. He neither longs for it nor fears it. It is only information. The warrior disregards concern for his own safety out of any fear of death. The idea of complete safety to the warrior is essentially an illusion. This is the mindset of a warrior, who commits energy to the fight at hand rather than to extraneous thoughts.

Commitment to something beyond oneself is a quality of the Samurai and many other warriors in history. Matthew 16:25 says, "That whoever wants to save his life will lose it, but whoever loses his life for [Jesus's] sake will find it." This scripture is opining about a spiritual relationship and many religions around the world contain similar ideas. Warriors possess this same mind-set about life and death. Being committed to something beyond one's own life has great value and leads one to put aside the fear of death.

Commitment involves both the heart and the mind. There is a story told by the ancient Roman writer Pliny the Elder (23–79 CE). He wrote about the raising of an obelisk that would stand 99 feet tall. Twenty thousand workers were selected to pull on the ropes that would hoist it. One small error would topple the structure and ruin years of work. The king insisted the engineer's own son be strapped to the top of the obelisk as it was hoisted so that the heart as well as the mind of the engineer would be committed to the task.[10]

To warriors such as the Samurai, the greatest tragedy was to lack principle. They would rather die than dishonor their names. Their minds and hearts were united in total commitment to the task at hand as result of this thinking.

It is difficult to defeat someone with this level of commitment. Be decisive and focused on a course of action without hesitation, then swiftly bring all forces to bear on that action. To win fights, one must be committed.

NOTES

1. Sun Tzu, *The Art of War and Other Classics of Eastern Thought* (New York: Barnes & Noble, 2013).
2. Sun Tzu, *Sun Tzu on the Art of War* (Gutenberg ebook Project: The British Museum, 1994), http://www.gutenberg.org/cache/epub/132/pg132-images .html.
3. BrainyQuote, "George Patton Quotes," https://www.brainyquote.com/quotes /quotes/g/georgespa138200.html.
4. UNCTV, "Cortes Burns His Boats," University of North Carolina Television, http://www.pbs.org/conquistadors/cortes/cortes_d00.html.
5. Corrie Ten Boom, "Wiseoldsayings," http://www.wiseoldsayings.com/authors /corrie-ten-boom-quotes/.
6. Yamamoto Tsunetomo, *Hagakure* (New York: Kodansha International, 1983).
7. The Physics Classroom, "Newton's Second Law," http://www.physicsclassroom .com/class/newtlaws/Lesson-3/Newton-s-Second-Law.
8. Miyamoto Musashi, *The Five Rings, Miyamoto Musashi's Art of Strategy: The New Illustrated Edition of the Japanese Warrior Classic* (New York: Quarto Publishing Group, 2012).
9. Inspirational Proverbs, Quotes, Sayings, "Latin Proverbs," http://www.inspi rationalstories.com/proverbs/latin-deliberate-often-decide-once/.
10. Bible.org, "Pliny the Elder," August 14, 1992, https://bible.org/illustration /pliny-elder.

致死性

リーダー武蔵

LETHALITY

"YOUR CONCENTRATION UPON destroying the enemy must be intense and single-minded," said Miyamoto Musashi (1584–1645).[1] As discussed, Musashi was a famous Samurai. He withdrew to a cave in order to meditate. While there he wrote *The Book of Five Rings*, which is a classic book on strategy. "Lethality" means to destroy or harm to whatever degree is sufficient to neutralize a threat. The U.S. armed forces define it as use of a force that could create substantial injury or risk of death.

No other word carries the complete range of necessary connotations. Lethality is the willingness to exert whatever force is necessary to win and includes the full range of possibilities. A lethal fighter is a dangerous fighter who will exert extreme aggression to win at all costs, doing whatever it takes and utilizing everything at his disposal. It is a misunderstood term.

A criminal does not fear a police officer because of his badge. He fears him because he carries a gun and is willing to use it. A vehicle has just as much lethal potential as a gun but isn't seen as lethal due to its nonlethal purpose. Let's merge these thoughts for a moment.

A warrior can be a gardener. His purpose in life is peaceful, just as a vehicle has the peaceful purpose of transportation. But a vehicle can be turned into a weapon or object of destruction in an instant, and a warrior must be able to become a weapon of destruction.

Musashi says an enemy must be destroyed in a fight. But civil society understands there are times when a threat may need to be neutralized rather than completely destroyed, such as the case of police subduing an offender. This requires levels of aggression.

Those who recoil at the thought of aggression as a tool necessary to win a fight view aggression like a gun, which is all or nothing. It is something many believe peacekeepers like police should not exhibit.

But there are varying degrees of aggression. There are varying degrees of intensity. There are varying levels of destructive power. Lethality is the willingness to embrace the entire range of ferocity needed to accomplish a task. While "destroy" is all or nothing, "lethality" embraces the idea that there is a wide range of options to neutralize a threat. But it also suggests there is no limit other than winning. That is why "destroy" may be too specific an idea and "aggressiveness" may be too broad.

An army can be aggressive. But are there limits to its aggression? Does it have strict rules of engagement? An animal may appear fierce. But is there a limit to its ferocity? Is the animal all bark and no bite? A police officer may be expected to serve and protect. But does he have self-imposed limits to how far he will go to protect? Do politicians handcuff his rules of engagement? Lethality implies there are no limits. A lethal fighter may be peaceful if needed. A lethal fighter may be extremely violent if needed.

Lethality can be proportional to how dangerous the fighter needs to be in a fight. While that scale of force may begin small, the end of the scale must have no limitation other than winning the fight. If a fighter has a limitation on how far he will go, then the opponent will go a bit farther and win. Limitations are what cause a fighter not to be lethal. Limitations on doing what it takes to win or neutralize a threat will cause a fighter to lose. Lethality creates a sense of unpredictability if an opponent does not know your limits.

If an army, an animal, or a police officer does not possess the ability to be lethal, which is the willingness to expend whatever aggression it takes to prevail, then there will be many who will not fear them. Because an enemy, predator, or criminal will simply exceed whatever limits are imposed in order to win. It makes defeating their prey simple: just be more lethal.

The one with the fewest restrictions in the fight has the greatest freedom to win. "Lethal" implies there are no restrictions.

If threatening individuals know they will be met by whatever level of lethality is necessary to stop them, then they will be afraid. Being lethal unfortunately means being willing to kill if necessary. Lethality has no limits and is a principle that can be controversial. But if enemies know you will crush them even if you have to kill them to save your own life, they will fear you. They will understand that you have no restrictions, no hesitation, and no aversion to doing what needs to be done. That is the essence of being lethal.

AGGRESSION

"Don't worry about your flanks. Let the enemy worry about his flanks," were the words of General George S. Patton (1885–1945). Patton was in a conference on August 1, 1944, with his officers when he made this observation.[2] He was commenting on the concept that flanks should be secured. Guarding the flanks had slowed many army advances. Patton said that before the enemy ever found out where his were located, he would have cut his enemy's throat.

Whether an ancient warrior or a modern-day general, the theme to winning is similar. In a fight, one must exhibit overwhelming aggression with a focus on destruction. The one who wins a fight is the most lethal or at least has the potential to be the most lethal. That fighter is generally the one that is most aggressive.

Musashi noted that the spirit of fire was fierce regardless of whether the flame was large or small. He correlated this fierceness to a quality needed to win fights. One must exert this fierce quality in battle. This is what makes a fighter lethal. It is the fighter's fierceness that emerges during a fight in order to win.

There is an old adage that the best defense is a good offense. An aggressive response to an attack often catches the attacker off guard. This overwhelming response is generally sufficient to put an end to any violence initiated by an attacker. A ruthless and aggressive response is the application of the principle of lethality.

Retired Lieutenant Colonel Dave Grossman is the world's foremost expert on human aggression. A former army ranger, Grossman is a psychology professor at West Point, the director of the Killology Research Group, and has written several books on aggression. *On Combat*, co-authored with Loren Christensen, investigates the psychology and physiology of deadly conflict in war and peace.

Grossman discusses the impact a few true warriors can have in battle. He quotes G. K. Chesterton, who said, "The paradox of courage is that a man must be a little careless of his life in order to keep it."[3] This is similar to the Samurai philosophy discussed earlier.

Grossman relates the perception held by many in regard to combat. In movies, for example, all the soldiers are intensely engaged in battle. But Grossman's statistics paint a different picture. His research reflects the Pareto principle that 20 percent of the people do 80 percent of the work in an organization. It is the law of the vital few.

S. L. A. Marshall was the U.S. Army's chief historian during World War II and the Korean War. Grossman relates Marshall's finding that the majority of soldiers in World War II never fired their weapons or at least didn't fire with the purpose of killing the enemy. Marshall's research indicated that between 75 and 85 percent of soldiers never fired their weapons. The work was a bit controversial at the time it was published and the methodology used to derive this number is often debated. But Marshall used the number to argue for more army training to increase the percentage of soldiers willing to engage the enemy in direct fire.

The Army isn't an organization that changes easily. But the research resulted in many changes in training. Only a few years later, the fire ratio in the Korean War had increased to over 50 percent. Marshall's influence is still felt as U.S. soldiers now are the highest trained force in the world. American forces are much more lethal today than during World War II as a result.

Grossman's overall point in using the figure is to relate how a few true warriors actually do most of the killing in combat. It's why World War II Medal of Honor recipient Charles "Commando" Kelly won the award. Though Grossman points out there were many other soldiers with Kelly when he pulled off his exploits, only one received the Medal of Honor.

Kelly killed 40 Germans in less than an hour and killed more the next day. He and 30 other soldiers were in a house surrounded by the enemy. Kelly used every weapon he could find in the house to fight back.[4] Again, he was not alone. There were other soldiers there as well. But he alone was more aggressive than the others. He was single-minded in his desire to destroy the enemy.

This demonstrates the lethality of a few men in combat. It is the Pareto principle applied to war: 80 percent of the outcomes are attributed to 20 percent of the causes. A few individuals can have a great impact. It is the 20 percent who are lethal.

The same principle is true in air warfare. A minority of aces succeeded in hitting the majority of enemy aircraft that were shot down. These pilots were able to accomplish these feats through their aggression and boldness of action.[5]

RESTRAINT

The problem with lethality is ambiguity. If you are a soldier faced with combat, there is little doubt about what you need to do. A soldier must go from zero to 100 percent lethal once immersed in combat. A soldier needs to be 100 percent lethal all the time while engaging the enemy. A soldier's job is simply to kill when in combat.

But if you are a police officer or other protector in a civilian role, your job is to protect, not kill. The level of lethality must be gauged to the situation. It should always match then just barely exceed the force necessary to overcome the situation. An officer or citizen must be just lethal enough to stop an attacker, but not any more than is necessary to neutralize the threat.

You may be forced to unfortunately kill in that role. You may be forced to be very aggressive to succeed in these civilian roles. But the level of lethality or aggression depends upon the force applied against your goal of self-preservation or protection. Killing the enemy isn't always the goal.

Unlike the soldier who has less doubt regarding the level of lethality required to do his job, noncombat situations require varying levels of lethality. A true warrior, regardless of whether the warrior is in combat or not, is willing to apply whatever lethality is necessary to neutralize a threat. It is the potential that makes a fighter lethal in those roles.

Again, legal experts always add that no force should be applied beyond what is necessary to neutralize the threat.[6] This is a sometimes ambiguous truth. But the attacker must at least know that the warrior is willing to apply whatever lethality is required without limits. A police officer must be diplomatic, patient, judicious, and prudent to neutralize violence. But he ultimately must have the potential to be totally lethal, otherwise he should not be carrying a gun, nor should anyone else if they are not willing to do whatever it takes to neutralize evil. A gun is a lethal weapon. If the person carrying the gun isn't willing to utilize the full potential of that lethal weapon, then the person is just taking a gun to a fight for someone else to use. Carrying a lethal weapon is not enough. The user must be willing to be lethal with it. A gun is simply a tool. It is the user that determines lethality.

The time to decide how lethal you can be is not during the heat of a battle. Warriors must decide in advance. Understand what the rules of engagement are for the situation, but understand that ultimately winning a fight may require varying levels of aggression to win and the most aggressive will prevail.

Firearms expert Jeff Cooper taught classes on these warrior principles. Many of his principles and gun fighting techniques were adopted by law enforcement agencies across the nation. But many rejected the principles of aggression he taught, as they seemed incongruent to peacekeepers. How can you tell peacekeepers to be aggressive in order to win fights but also keep the peace?[7]

This is why lethality is probably a better description. It is possible to be too aggressive. Sun Tzu advised using deception to lure an aggressive army into a trap. He explained that holding out bait, such as feigning disorder, would entice aggressive armies and then crush them.[8] Aggression must be tempered by discipline. Lethality implies a two-way street with a path to either escalation or deescalation of force.

While it is true that the most aggressive typically wins fights, it is with the caveat that the fighter who knows how to focus aggression properly will win the fight. Discipline is the throttle of aggression.

Peacekeepers must understand this paradox. It doesn't mean they must be aggressive in every situation. A fight may not even occur if the enemy knows the peacekeeper is at least potentially lethal. Aggression and lethality are two different things but the same thing in this paradox. Aggression is the vehicle that delivers lethality. It isn't enough for the enemy to know you are aggressive. You must be lethal. You must be willing to do anything to win. This is why sometimes simply producing a weapon in an altercation stops the altercation. The lethal potential of the weapon overrides everything else.

FLIPPING THE SWITCH

We once trained a martial artist who was great in the dojo. He had more skill and aptitude than anyone. His technique was flawless. But he never won in a full contact mixed martial arts match. It wasn't his technique that was the problem. His will was the problem.

He was fast, he was powerful, and his timing and technique were superb. But he was also a terribly nice guy. Now there is nothing wrong with being a nice guy. But when you enter a cage fight with few rules, the nice guy attitude must be replaced with ferocity. The fighter must be lethal in the cage. Fighters call it flipping a switch in their brain.

Once the fight is on, the nice guy mind-set cannot be in the cage. The aggressively lethal mind-set must be in the cage.

LETHAL COMPONENTS

The definition of "lethal" has a couple of components in terms of intensity. One component is the capacity to cause death. If an officer is not capable of this, then he is dangerous to himself as there are limits to how much he can or will protect.

In *Deadly Force Encounters*, authors Loren Christiansen and Dr. Alexis Artwohl relate a paintball test once given to veteran officers in Nebraska.[9] The officers were given the scenario of "officer needs help with shots fired."

When the officer arrived at the simulated scenario he found a suspect standing over a downed officer. The suspect points at the officer, yelling he is going to kill the downed officer. The uneasy part is that the suspect has his back to the arriving officer.

In the scenario, the authors say that the majority of officers would not fire. They fired only after the suspect shot the downed officer. A significant number fired only after the suspect pointed his weapon at them and many times the reaction time was so delayed that the arriving officer was shot as well. It wasn't an action that saved innocent lives. If the officer doesn't know how to flip the switch, the officer isn't lethal. Training and discipline help guide when to flip the switch.

The other component of lethality is to be extremely harmful or devastating. It is lower intensity than the component capable of killing. This is the component of lethality that applies to something like our friend, the cage fighter who is a nice guy but couldn't be lethal in terms of being devastating in the cage because his nice guy attitude was in the cage with him limiting his ability to be lethal to the necessary level to win. He needed to beat the opponent and trust his discipline to tell him when to stop, as winning the fight is the goal, not killing the opponent.

Our nice guy fighter wasn't raised in an environment that required development of certain survival instincts. He hadn't trained for situations where his mental attitude must shift dramatically, so his opponent had the mental edge. A fighter must know how to flip that mental switch. If he isn't willing to be devastating then he holds something back. He isn't lethal. Being lethal is holding nothing back when the time comes to fight. But that level of brutality can be gauged with discipline until aggression is needed to deliver it when a fight does begin.

Which returns us to the words of the Samurai Musashi, who said that concentration on destroying the enemy must be intense and single-minded. These recurring principled themes occur throughout the martial arts literature. To win a fight, a fighter must possess the full potential of lethality and be willing to deliver whatever it takes to win.

In a civil society, life is given priority over property. And every fight doesn't or shouldn't end with the death of the opponent. Being lethal is to possess potential force that should be gauged depending on the situation. This potential for being dangerous must be ever present and match the level of aggression needed to win the fight. Matching means to deliver a disciplined amount of aggression to overcome the opponent.

Aggression, Lethality, and Peace

Psychologist Steven Pinker wrote about violence from an altruistic perspective in his book *The Better Angels of Our Nature*.[10] He tried to make the point that violence has decreased in modern times. It is a statistical stretch and a difficult construct to measure. His book was a best seller. Critics such as writer John Gray say this is wishful thinking. Gray is an author and Emeritus Professor of European Thought at the London School of Economics and a regular contributor to *The Guardian* newspaper. Gray calls the figures murky and notes there is no reason to think man is becoming more altruistic or peaceful.[11]

There is a notion that the spread of capitalism and globalization accounts for fewer war fatalities as war can be costly by disrupting trade, but then again war can be profitable in some quarters as well. So that isn't entirely an answer to changing fatality numbers noted by Pinker.

Also, you have to understand how nations collect data about war fatalities. It wasn't an accurate exercise in ancient times, plus there were far fewer people, thus percentages can be deceiving. Even today military contractors such as Blackwater USA and other groups are not included in government war fatality numbers. Current wars owe a huge debt to these contractors, yet they are considered expendable and are invisible to nations.[12]

John Lott's book *More Guns, Less Crime*[13] presents specific figures that show a decrease in violent crime in areas where concealed carry laws are passed. He cites more than 29 years of data for every county in the United States. His research supports the idea that principles such as the potential to be lethal are deterrents to crime and result in less violence. Steven Pinker would probably cringe at the thought that his conclusions of less violence could be the result of John Lott's conclusions. Lott makes the point that guns may be one reason crime has decreased or that we've become more efficient at delivering violence, making violence less tenable. Wars are more efficient as well. Technology permits more focused targeting of the enemy. Civilian casualties are more limited as a result. Yet armies have more destructive potential than ever before.

Whether violence is on the rise or decline is a matter of perspective and which data you'd like to read. But it is clear that man has always been violent and is actually getting better at it. There is no evidence it is in significant enough decline that we should let our guard down. I recall that when I was a boy we left our doors unlocked. No one would think that is a good idea today.

The statistical odds of being in a fight are suddenly 100 percent once you are involved in it, and no one should believe they are immune to violence. The nature of man has always been one of violence. It isn't man who has changed, but the tools with which he wages war and the statistical methods he uses to measure conflict have evolved. In the end, what do you do with the information from Pinker or Lott? Regardless of whose numbers you believe, you should still remain alert, as it is not wise to do anything else.

The adage that an armed society is a polite society is true. You hear about the Wild West but gun laws were even stricter during the time of the OK Corral. After all, that's the reason Wyatt Earp got in his famous shootout enforcing Tombstone gun laws, which didn't work too well because only thugs carried guns.[14]

Human aggression is complex and evil people willing to exert violence will always exist. These evil people will also ignore laws and any sense of civility. It takes the equalizing nature of lethality to combat this violence in whatever data set you wish to measure it.

Disciplined Aggression

Distinguishing between aggression and lethality is important. I've described lethality as the power to exert whatever force is necessary to win, including lethal force if necessary. We've also noted that the most aggressive fighter will win and that aggression should be disciplined to overcome the opponent. But there is a downside to aggression without discipline.

Overly aggressive fighters are simply bullies. They are easy targets and essentially beat themselves, as uncontrolled aggression creates blind spots. An overly aggressive fighter responds to the tempo of a fight but doesn't control it. An aggressive fighter who is disciplined will control the tempo. If a fighter controls the tempo of the fight, he is fighting his own fight rather than letting his opponent control the fight. Disciplined aggression that controls the tempo of action is a winning skill.

I see this issue repeat itself constantly at ringside as a boxing commissioner, whether it's a boxing match or a mixed martial arts event. There are fighters with great skills and enormous aggression. They are lethal. But they fail to control the tempo and essentially beat themselves when faced with a more disciplined fighter.

Don't confuse aggression with anger. Sigmund Freud said, "Anger leads to fear, fear leads to hate, and hate leads to the dark side."[15] You can be angry with someone without being aggressive. You can also be aggressive but not angry. Aggression is a behavior while anger is an emotion. Both need to be controlled and focused.

Force should be limited to gain compliance or win in a fight. Then force is withdrawn. But it is anger that may cause someone to use force beyond what is necessary. Differentiating the two is all about discipline, which is a requirement to have lethal results and to use lethality responsibly.

In *Tools of Titans*, Tim Ferriss describes someone who has a fitness goal of doing one push-up every day.[16] Now he knows once he does one, he is going to do more. But it's how he disciplines himself to get started.

Motivation is great. You may be motivated to exercise. But it takes discipline to actually do it. Discipline gets things started while motivation is fleeting. Discipline is doing whatever it takes every day.

If a fighter understands how to deliver significant injury or even death but also has the discipline to control that devastation, then the fighter has what is called lethal leverage.

In the dojo, we have black belts spar with the new white belts that are sparring for the first time so no one gets hurt. New fighters do not know how to control a fight. They do not know their own strength. Accidents happen.

Black belts know how to control the whole spectrum of their skill. The black belt can self-protect and keep the novice from doing any unintended damage during sparring. If a fighter knows how to deliver maximum bodily injury upon an opponent, then the fighter also knows how not to deliver it. But a new fighter has no idea when to stop or start. Novices don't know their strength.

My first instructor was Master Nathaniel Thompson. He was a Professional Karate Association full contact state champion. He would have us control our blows while training. He always said that if you can control a punch or kick and stop it just as it made contact, then you could take the opponent's head off if you wanted to. It was all about control, but you had to know the full range of possibilities to achieve this control. Control wins over brute force. As a side note, when asked by students how hard should they hit when sparring in class, his answer was to hit as hard as you want to be hit. It's always about controlling force and discipline.

There is simply a difference between brute force and lethal efficiency. Brute force doesn't take much thinking or control. It is the difference between a fighter trying to win by muscle not knowing how to control or focus anything and a professional who knows the full range of his capabilities. At ringside, you can tell the professional fighter from the newer fighter who tries to win simply by using brute force abilities. The disciplined professional wins nearly every time.

Much of lethality is simply mind-set. It is a mind-set of winning at all costs and a valuable principle. If a fighter is lethal and aggressive, then the fighter is essentially unstoppable.

NOTES

1. Miyamoto Musashi, *The Five Rings, Miyamoto Musashi's Art of Strategy: The New Illustrated Edition of the Japanese Warrior Classic* (New York: Quarto Publishing Group, 2012).
2. Stanley Hirshon, *General Patton: A Soldier's Life* (New York: Harper Perennial, 2003).
3. Dave Grossman and Loren Christensen, *On Combat: The Psychology and Physiology of Deadly Conflict in War and Peace* (Mascoutah, IL: Warrior Science Publications, 2008).
4. Duane Schultz, "'Commando' Charles Kelly and the First European Theater Medal of Honor," *Warfare History Network* (December 3, 2014), http://warfare historynetwork.com/daily/wwii/commando-charles-kelly-the-first-european -theater-medal-of-honor/.
5. Phillip Kaplan, *Fighter Aces of the Luftwaffe in World War II* (South Yorkshire, UK: Pen and Sword, 2007).
6. Graham v. Connor, 490 U.S. 386 (1989), https://supreme.justia.com/cases/federal /us/490/386/.
7. Timothy Williams, "Long Taught to Use Force, Police Warily Learn to De-escalate," *New York Times*, June 28, 2015, A16.

8. Sun Tzu, *The Art of War and Other Classics of Eastern Thought* (New York: Barnes & Noble, 2013).

9. Loren Christensen and Alexis Artwohl, *Deadly Force Encounters: What Cops Need to Know to Mentally and Physically Prepare for and Survive a Gunfight* (Boulder, CO: Paladin Press, 1997).

10. Steven Pinker, *The Better Angels of Our Nature: Why Violence Has Declined* (New York: Penguin, 2012).

11. John Gray, "Steven Pinker Is Wrong about Violence and War," *Guardian*, March 13, 2015, https://www.theguardian.com/books/2015/mar/13/john-gray-steven-pinker-wrong-violence-war-declining.

12. Ed Hiner, "Unsung Heroes, Not 'Mercenaries,'" *San Diego Union-Tribune*, June 11, 2017, http://www.sandiegouniontribune.com/military/guest-voices/sd-me-hiner-contractors-20170607-story.html.

13. John Lott, *More Guns, Less Crime: Understanding Crime and Gun Control Laws* (Chicago: University of Chicago Press, 2010).

14. Bob Drogin, "Gun Laws Were Tougher in Old Tombstone," *Los Angeles Times*, January 23, 2011, http://articles.latimes.com/2011/jan/23/nation/la-na-tombstone-20110123.

15. Paul Joseph, *The SAGE Encyclopedia of War: Social Sciences Perspectives* (Thousand Oaks, CA: SAGE Publications, 2016), 770.

16. Tim Ferriss, *Tools of Titans* (New York: Houghton Mifflin Harcourt, 2017).

効率性

リーダー武蔵

EFFICIENCY

EFFICIENCY ENCOMPASSES a couple of concepts: speed and economy of motion. They are interrelated.

General George Patton said, "A good solution applied with vigor now, is better than a perfect solution applied ten minutes later."[1] He echoed Sun Tzu's observation centuries earlier: "Be swift . . . fast as lightning that flashes before you can blink your eyes."[2]

The efficiency of the fighter, in terms of speed and economy of motion, will essentially determine the fight's outcome. Being lethal is of little consequence if focus and aggression are not applied quickly and with vigor while maximizing energy. Actions must be efficient.

Miyamoto Musashi recognized that swift application of an attack is more than just speed. Something can be done fast but be terribly inefficient. He believed in quickness and agility when describing speed.[3] Bruce Lee reflected this concept in his teachings of no wasted motion.

The military has a saying that slow is smooth and smooth is fast. It is a particularly popular view among snipers. Motion should be quick but not reckless. It should be swift and deliberate. These are the mechanics behind efficiency.

Remember, every passing second in a conflict favors the attacker. Almost every text on combat recommends a swift end to conflict. A perfect fight is one that has ended before your opponent realizes what is happening.

There are caveats to nearly every principle. The first part of efficiency certainly is speed and a swift end to conflict is the optimal model. However, speed isn't always the best economy of motion. Speed is simply the first option. If it were the only option then speed itself would be the principle. Being fast for the sake of being fast isn't the only consideration.

Economy of Motion

When faced with a stronger enemy it is often more economical to retreat. You buy space with time, as time is more important than space. In this context, it is the retreat that is quick and deliberate. This is the motion of efficiency: executing action that expends the least amount of energy but achieves the greatest advantage or effect is the core concept of efficiency. Efficiency is about the utilization of:

1. Speed
2. Time
3. Space

The I-Ching is an eighth-century Chinese document in which it is written that an orderly retreat is the only correct strategy if faced with a superior force with which engagement would be hopeless.[4]

Napoleon Bonaparte said that he could recover space. But he couldn't recover time.[5] If creating space is the needed strategy in a fight, then it should be done speedily. Once space has been managed, an attack can be planned when the conditions are right. Attacks and retreats should both be accomplished efficiently.

The key is to end the conflict before the opponent is aware of what is happening. But this only applies if engagement is the decided course of action. You do not want to win a battle but lose the war. Efficiency, and not each of its separate components (time, space, speed), is the overriding principle. Decide what action is most efficient, apply it quickly, vigorously, and with the most economic use of motion.

Pick your battles and be swift in the execution of each battle. Make the opponent fight your fight. This is the most efficient use of force and resources.

The Arab-Israeli Six-Day War is a tactical example. When faced with overwhelming opposition, the Israelis essentially had no means to retreat, as the country is small. When threatened by neighboring countries they quickly launched offensive actions and caught their enemies off guard. The war was short. They defeated many countries in a few days, ending the threat. Fewer than a thousand Israelis were killed. The countries they opposed lost around 20,000.[6]

This contrasts with Vietnam. Guerrilla troops would strike South Vietnamese targets quickly then retreat, even though American forces protecting the South were much more powerful. The Vietcong never wanted a fair fight. They fought the fight with which they were most comfortable, as they knew they would lose a traditional fight against the stronger U.S. forces. The Vietcong used efficient principles against American forces fighting their fight instead. The Vietcong prolonged the conflict to their advantage while stateside politicians interfered with warriors' plans on the ground. The Vietnamese guerrilla tactics had no rules. But traditional U.S. military planners had many rules of engagement placed on them by politicians. This put efficiency in the hands of the Vietcong.

The same guerrilla strategies were utilized by colonists against British forces during the Revolutionary War. American forces were more efficient in their use of force.

RIGHT FOCUS

Efficiency isn't just doing something right, but doing the right things. Doing the right things is performing useful work to achieve a goal rather than action that is an inefficient use of energy.

In 2004, General Stanley A. McChrystal commanded the Joint Special Operations Command in Iraq. He had the best forces in the world and could win any battle. His problem was that new terrorists were still emerging everywhere. His problem was not force capability, but efficiency.

Intelligence derived from raids or interrogations took time to be analyzed. By the time military planners assessed the information it was no longer actionable as it had to be passed along many lines before reaching those who needed it to make decisions.

General McChrystal had a great force that operated perfectly and was quite lethal. But network designs prevented efficient application of that force. Individual principles such as lethality must be coupled with other principles in order to win fights. Just having a lethal force isn't enough. Efficient application of that force is necessary.

In the civilian world, a manager would have tried to bring in consultants and redesign jobs. But General McChrystal recognized that the problem was not in how the soldiers did their job. They did it well. It was a problem of efficient vision of the overall mission. Each unit, from raiding teams to intelligence officers, did their jobs and knew what to do. But the network that linked those jobs was inefficient.

The general empowered the ground troops by redesigning command and control structures. He embedded intelligence analysts with raiding teams and ensured constant interaction between systems. They then had the resources to respond more quickly to intelligence. Rather than just performing a job they were provided the ability to see the whole system.[7]

Having a strong army or a great plan is fine. But either is worthless if you don't have an efficient means to deploy the army or accomplish the plan.

Efficiency was a problem in Mogadishu, Somalia. In 1993, Special Operators tried to rescue soldiers in a downed Black Hawk helicopter.[8] Some recalled later that the reason they got lost on the complex streets was due to a delay in getting directions from spotters overhead. Aircraft would tell operators to turn right on the next street attempting to guide them to the downed helicopter, but by the time the information was relayed they had traveled several blocks. Information transfer was inefficient.

In yet another example of inefficiency, some swimmers try to pound the water using force to generate momentum. The problem is they create waves, which results in more water resistance. An efficient swimmer keeps the water smooth in front of them, moving steadily but only as fast as the water allows. The swimmer doesn't fight the water but works with it. In the end, the efficient swimmer covers the most distance.

There is a fable about a goose and a horse. The goose proudly tells the horse that a goose is nobler than a horse because a goose inhabits three elements. A goose can fly, swim, or walk on dry land. A horse is confined to land, as a horse cannot fly and does not inhabit the water.

The horse replies that although this is true, the horse is a far nobler creature. The horse commands the ground it inhabits. The horse is powerful and swift.

The horse says that although the goose indeed inhabits three elements it makes no distinguishing mark on any of them. In the air a goose is no match for an eagle or even a sparrow. The goose is heavy and flies clumsily through the air compared to other birds.

In the water, a goose that swims on the surface cannot be compared to a fish that lives there. A goose is no match for a fish in terms of efficient swimming.

On dry land a goose waddles when trying to walk. Its feet are broad and movement is slow. A goose certainly inhabits three elements but does not efficiently inhabit any of them in comparison to other creatures.[9]

Daniel Goleman relates a striking example of efficiency in his book *Emotional Intelligence*. Goleman describes the experience of an aikido martial artist friend.[10] Aikido is a very complex martial art and focuses on efficiency of movement. There is much philosophy associated with the art.

Goleman relates that his aikido friend was one of the first Westerners to train under aikido's founder, Morihei Ueshiba. His friend was on a subway in the 1960s during his time training at the Hombu dojo in Tokyo when a very large drunk man stepped on the train.

The drunk began harassing everyone and tension was rising. The American aikido student said he was already planning how he could use his aikido techniques to neutralize the large man.

But just before the American martial artist was about to spring into action, a small elderly Japanese man stood up between the large drunk and the American. The old man began speaking calmly to the much larger drunk. He explained how he understood the drunk knowing life must be hard for him.

Before the American realized it, the drunk was crying in the old man's lap. It was at that moment the American realized he had witnessed true aikido efficiency in action and had a lot to learn. The old man had subdued and controlled the drunk with words alone.

EFFICIENCY AND EFFECTIVENESS

The difference between efficiency and effectiveness must also be understood. Efficiency is determined by resource utilization. It is the ratio of work conducted in relation to the resources supplied. To be efficient, the maximum attainable work is accomplished with the fewest resources or least amount of energy.

Effectiveness is the ratio between actual and theoretical accomplishment.[11] It is a comparison of potential output and actual output. It really tells us nothing about efficiency, as the term "productivity" is the ratio between efficiency and effectiveness. Productivity is another measure in this regard. Effectiveness is an outcome.

If the intended result is accomplished, then the process is effective, although there are varying degrees of effectiveness just as there are varying degrees of efficiency. The action may have been effective but by inefficient means.

Efficiency may increase the chances of effectiveness though effectiveness otherwise has little relationship to efficiency. It's a bit of an academic point but hopefully provides clarity to these terms, which are often used interchangeably.

EFFICIENCY WINS FIGHTS

Efficiency is the swift and economical use of resources. An efficient method must be effective as well, thus accomplishing the intended purpose.

Bruce Lee said that "efficiency is anything that scores."[12] Efficiency is using what works and what is at your disposal. A high spinning kick looks nice. It may be effective, but it isn't necessarily efficient. But a quick strike to an attacker's throat is efficient as well as effective. It also swiftly ends conflict.

Gary Keller is an entrepreneur and author. His book, *The One Thing*, has some extraordinary truths on efficiency. He asks, "What is the one thing you can do such that by doing it everything else will be easier or unnecessary?"[13] The question is the essence of efficiency. He adds that focus is deciding what things you are not going to do. Focus and efficiency are closely related concepts.

Efficiency, effectiveness, and focus are common themes in winning a fight quickly. Ending conflict without any wasted motion or by the utilization of the least amount of energy is efficiency. And while effectiveness can be more objectively measured, efficiency is better viewed as a percentage of input used to achieve the result.

Again, the Pareto principle is a good example of this measure. Sometimes called the 80/20 rule, it states that 80 percent of the effects come from 20 percent of the cause. Have you ever noticed that 20 percent of the people in an organization seem to be the ones that do 80 percent of the work? That's the Pareto principle in action.

Pareto showed that about 80 percent of the land in Italy was owned by 20 percent of the population.[14] He developed his principle after noting 20 percent of his peapods in his garden contained 80 percent of the peas. In business, it has been noted that 80 percent of sales come from 20 percent of clients. The list goes on, but it is clear how efficiency impacts effectiveness.

It is easy to see that efficiency allows a small percentage to have a great impact. That is the reason efficiency is a principle, as fighters must execute actions by the best means to achieve results. The efficient use of force is generally the best and isn't determined by size. It is determined by speed and economy of motion.

Notes

1. Stanley Hirshon, *General Patton: A Soldier's Life* (New York: Harper Perennial, 2003).
2. Sun Tzu, *The Art of War and Other Classics of Eastern Thought* (New York: Barnes & Noble, 2013).
3. Miyamoto Musashi, *The Five Rings, Miyamoto Musashi's Art of Strategy: The New Illustrated Edition of the Japanese Warrior Classic* (New York: Quarto Publishing Group, 2012).
4. King Wen, *I-Ching* (1899), https://archive.org/details/I-Ching.
5. Military Quotes, "Napoleon Bonaparte," http://www.military-quotes.com /Napoleon.htm.
6. Mitchell Bard, "The Six-Day War: Background and Overview," *Jewish Virtual Library* (2008), http://www.jewishvirtuallibrary.org/background-and-overview -six-day-war.

7. Loren Mooney, "Gen. Stanley McChrystal: Adapt to Win in the 21st Century," *Stanford Business* (April 15, 2014), https://www.gsb.stanford.edu/insights/gen-stanley-mcchrystal-adapt-win-21st-century.

8. Richard Stewart, *The US Army in Somalia* (2002), http://www.history.army.mil/brochures/Somalia/Somalia.htm.

9. Darren Poke, "The Goose and the Horse—A Story about Maximizing Your Strengths," Better Life Coaching Blog, October 19, 2012, https://betterlifecoachingblog.com/2012/10/19/the-goose-and-the-horse-a-story-about-maximising-your-strengths/.

10. Daniel Goleman, *Emotional Intelligence* (New York: Random House, 2012).

11. Vivek Saxena, "How to Calculate Effective Capacity and Efficiency," *Sciencing* (2017), http://sciencing.com/calculate-effective-capacity-efficiency-10067450.html.

12. Bruce Lee, *The Tao of Jeet Kune Do* (Santa Clarita, CA: Ohara, 1975).

13. Gary Keller, *The One Thing: The Surprisingly Simple Truth behind Extraordinary Results* (Austin, TX: Bard Press, 2013).

14. Dave Lavinsky, "Pareto Principle: How to Use It to Dramatically Grow Your Business," *Forbes*, January 20, 2014, https://www.forbes.com/sites/davelavinsky/2014/01/20/pareto-principle-how-to-use-it-to-dramatically-grow-your-business/#29b67c7e3901.

自制心

リーダー 武蔵

DISCIPLINE

ONE OF MY TEACHERS frequently used the phrase, "Keep a cool tool." Samurai Miyamoto Musashi expressed this a bit more eloquently centuries earlier, saying, "You must remain calm at all times; in this way you can control the attack."[1]

Lack of control is inefficient. A fighter must not lose composure. Controlled anger is fine, but control is the defining element, as controlled emotions like anger can be focused for maximum efficiency. You can see how the principles begin to come together.

Lt. Col. Jeff Cooper referred to a principle he called coolness.[2] Cooper was a U.S. Marine who served during World War II and the Korean War. He founded the American Pistol Institute, which later became known as Gunsite Academy in Arizona. He is credited with developing the modern technique of shooting, which is a two-handed stance rather than one-handed shooting. He is the author of numerous works and taught gun fighting technique.

He agreed anger was not an obstacle to efficiency as long as it was controlled. He also noted that self-control was something a sociopath does not possess. Most opponents or enemies do not possess self-control, so coolness is not a bad way to view discipline. In the balance of things, failure to be calm and disciplined under violent threat can have deadly consequences.

On April 5, 1970, a gunfight left four California Highway Patrol (CHP) officers dead in Newhall, California. The incident has been credited with initiating the police officer survival movement, and has been recounted in many law enforcement journals.[3]

Around 40 shots were fired in the firefight. Several shots were 12-gauge buckshot rounds from CHP officers that inflicted only one superficial wound on their assailants. The firefight lasted four minutes at a range of under 7 yards. It occurred at night making visibility poor.

There are many factors that favor attackers and sociopaths, such as having the element of surprise on their side in most instances and poor lighting conditions as in the Newhall incident. These elements may have factored into the shooting outcome with the CHP officers.

It should not be marksmanship that resulted in the death of the CHP troopers that night, but there have been questions about familiarity with their weapons and reloading them since the incident. Quite a few changes to police procedures and training were initiated as a result.

Allowing for all the other variables that resulted in poor marksmanship at such close range in the 1970 incident, it was ultimately the loss of concentration that affected the outcome. Under stressful firing conditions, the troopers lost their cool and were outgunned by focused killers whose fire was more disciplined. According to an assessment by Massad Ayoob, one trooper was killed before he was able to fire a shot. Another fired once before being killed. The third trooper fired six shots and was killed before he could reload his revolver. The last trooper fired three rounds from his shotgun, inadvertently ejected a fourth round, and fired four from his revolver before he was killed. But this isn't a rare incident.[4] Missing at close range during stress firing conditions occurs more often than you'd expect.

Although police departments routinely train officers up to 25 yards on a firing range, most gunfights occur in fewer than 10 yards. The hit ratio at such a close range is remarkably low.

In one New York Police Department study of gunfights between 1994 and 2000, officers' hit ratio was 38 percent at fewer than 2 yards. At 3 to 7 yards it drops to 17 percent and 8 to 15 yards 9 percent. These are trained officers and many factors contribute to the low ratios. But the overriding variable is disciplined fire, as there is growing evidence that training under low light conditions and stress fire situations helps improve these numbers.

Fast-forward to the present day with officers who have many years of experience with updated training techniques to achieve discipline under stress. One such officer escaped national news by not firing rather than utilizing disciplined fire. An incident makes national news only when an officer gets it wrong or someone is killed. Discipline under stress has proven to be effective in many modern instances despite the media spotlight given to select cases.

Off-duty law enforcement officer Burnis Wilkins was at home when he heard shots nearby. He then saw a young man running toward him. Wilkins accessed a weapon and ordered the man to stop. The man, who was carrying a handgun, began to run away from Wilkins.

Wilkins gave chase. Upon reaching an obstacle the young man spun around. Wilkins noticed the slide was locked back on the man's weapon, which meant it was jammed or out of ammunition. Though some say it was still a risky move, Wilkins held his fire and apprehended the suspect, who had allegedly just fired the weapon, wounding others.[5]

Imagine the discipline under stress that Wilkins's actions required. He put himself at great risk, but this officer practiced what he taught others as a law enforcement instructor. Discipline and "coolness under pressure" can be achieved with training and practice.

DISCIPLINE UNDER PRESSURE

We probably can attribute about 30 percent of our susceptibility to anxiety to DNA, according to a study among twins.[6] But that still doesn't mean we can't control that 30 percent, which leaves a lot of room for outside influences to impact how cool we are under pressure.

Boston Celtic player Bill Russell routinely became so nervous before games he would throw up.[7] But he was always cool under pressure during games. Anxiety may be a factor regarding performance, but it is clear that many control the correlation while others do not.

British Officer Lionel Wigram led one of the earliest studies to examine this phenomenon. In 1943, he noticed that each time his 22-man platoon encountered enemy fire his men responded in the same manner. A few reacted coolly and returned fire. Fewer would panic and try to escape. But the vast majority would freeze, unsure what to do.[8]

Survival psychologist John Leach studied a random group of people who found themselves in a sudden disaster, such as a fire. He noted similar results to Wigram's earlier observations. About 10 to 20 percent stayed calm, the majority (about 80 percent) were dazed and hesitant, and about 10 to 15 percent panicked. Leach refers to this as the 10-80-10 theory.[9]

Keep in mind that in 1943 the training of soldiers was nowhere near current-day training. Contemporary training methods have shown that realistic training conditions improve discipline under fire.

In the civilian world, simple fire drills improve responsiveness to these emergencies and increase coolness under pressure. But again, many people stand around seeking more information. Information improves discipline.[10]

Well-disciplined people who function well under stress share certain core beliefs:[11]

1. They see uncertainty as an opportunity and not as something dangerous.
2. Under stress their focus is on how to improve the situation.
3. They maintain a sense of commitment instead of withdrawing helplessly.

Interviews with people who have been involved in stressful situations yet maintained their composure reveal that all of them felt a level of fear. So keeping cool isn't the absence of fear. In many cases fear even helped fuel their response. It is the ability to focus fear into productive activity that makes the difference. This disciplined approach to functioning under pressure trains the mind to avoid being driven by distractions during stressful moments.

Disciplined training produces a specific pattern of behavior or character. Discipline is structured behavior that enhances improved actions both physically and mentally. Drills, constructive punishment, rewards, goal setting, and otherwise practicing a code of behavior under certain conditions improve reactions to situations. Discipline has the power to shape character.

Taekwondo legend Jhoon Rhee contends that discipline could solve many of society's problems aside from just winning fights. In an article published twice in *Black Belt Magazine*, Rhee says that people are a product of education. If they are taught to be communist, they become communist. If they are taught to be liars, they lie. But if they are taught to be honest, they are honest. He says why not teach discipline? Rhee believes teaching students the virtues of hard work, honesty, and respect is the solution to many of society's issues.[12]

Master Ummon was a zen master during the T'ang dynasty in China around 864–949 CE. He once said that, "if you walk, just walk. If you sit, just sit. But whatever you do, don't wobble."[13] His point was to always be disciplined and poised. It was rare for a Samurai to succumb to passion or emotion. A Samurai was not known to ever lose his cool. Whether walking or fighting, a Samurai maintained a sense of discipline to a poised pattern of behavior and character. Discipline is simply the ability to do what is necessary regardless of whether it is convenient.

In the movie *The Last Samurai*,[14] the character Captain Nathan Algren embraces the Samurai culture after being hired to destroy them. He makes this transition after being captured and held by the Samurai in their village.

Algren notes that from the moment the Samurai awake, they devote themselves totally to the perfection of whatever they pursue. Even in the most trivial moments of their day, they show great devotion to the task at hand. He says he has never seen such discipline and is surprised that the word "Samurai" means to serve. The movie depicts how the Samurai pursue greatness in even routine daily activities, pursuing perfection in everything they do through disciplined action.

Today, many want to be great but fail to act in a disciplined way to pursue greatness. Pursuing greatness is an active daily process achieved through small steps of self-discipline every day and revealed in even trivial moments. Discipline then becomes a habit by incorporating self-discipline in daily activities.

Doubt creates a disconnection between intent and action. This is why the Samurai were so devoted and focused on everything they did. It is why discipline is so important as a principle of fighting. In a fight, a

Samurai knew that a moment of doubt or unfocused attention during a time when his opponent had no doubt and was more focused could mean defeat. Intense focus on the most mundane daily activities creates the discipline to focus on everything else.

DISCIPLINED FIGHTING

Samurai disciplined themselves to fight smart. Their goal was to win at all cost.

Lt. Col. Jeff Cooper is often quoted but didn't say that "if you find yourself in a fair fight, your tactics suck." He more specifically said that it is actually the goal of the tactician (fighter) to ensure that the fight is never fair.[15]

The earliest example of this concept is again the Samurai Musashi. Once another great warrior named Sasaki Kojiro challenged him. Kojiro was known for using a slightly longer sword that gave him a reach advantage. It was harder to wield but he won many of his duels with this long sword, which made him a feared warrior.

Musashi showed up to the duel three hours late. His tardiness was meant to frustrate Kojiro. It also allowed for the sun to be lower on the horizon.

The duel was scheduled to occur on a beach. Musashi arrived with the sun at his back. Kojiro was already waiting on the beach, facing the sun.

Knowing Kojiro would have a longer sword than what was usually carried by warriors, Musashi left his own sword behind and cut off the head of the oar he had used to paddle to the beach as he was arriving by water.

He would use the oar as a bokken or wooden practice sword. It was sturdy but light and much longer than Kojiro's sword. Holding a longer weapon but one that was easier to maneuver was a clever tactic. Musashi now had many advantages, which created an unfair fight. Musashi won.[16] I am convinced that if Musashi were alive today, he would embrace gun fighting or any other superior method or tool to win.

The Samurai disciplined themselves not to be ruled by their own petty emotions. They focused on the perfection of everything they did. They might carry a book when not practicing with their sword or martial art. They may focus intently on other pursuits such as gardening. But they were disciplined in every task.

When studying the art of fighting, they approached winning the fight with discipline and examined everything that it would take to win the fight and execute those actions. They were composed at all times, including times of duress.

During the time of the Samurai there were few laws. The Samurai were so honorable and self-disciplined few laws were needed. Their personal code was clearly defined. Honorable men are always men of discipline. No one must force honorable men to do the right thing as they will do the right thing even when no one is watching. This is part of the warrior code.

Discipline is all about the journey. When studying martial arts, no instructor is going to set the highest goal first. Each step is taken in sequence, one at a time. Have you noticed the higher-ranking students in a karate class stand in front of lower-ranking ones? It's not simply a construct of hierarchy. It has a practical purpose. The reason is that a student only needs to observe the student standing in front of him or her to understand the next goal in skill level that needs to be achieved.

Small goals are attained and are then followed by increasingly higher goals. Discipline means focusing energy each step of the way.

CONTROLLED DISCIPLINE

If winning were about strength alone, then the larger opponent would always win. Discipline is about control and a strategy that is as important as strength. Incessant practice increases discipline, which becomes strength itself. Practice develops discipline so that discipline becomes a habit.

Navy Admiral William McRaven, a former Navy Seal, explained in a commencement speech at the University of Texas, Austin, that the best way to start the day was to make your bed. He said it provides a sense of pride and you've accomplished the first task of the day. This provides the discipline to accomplish another task and another task as the day progresses. Incessant action produces discipline and develops confidence. It is what is meant by a controlled, step-wise approach. Doing so creates a lasting habit that is stronger than motivation alone.[17]

The development of discipline among warriors has remained the same for centuries. From the ancient Samurai to Navy Seals, these warriors understand how attention to detail in every task develops a disciplined character.

MOTIVATION OR DISCIPLINE

Be careful about motivation. Motivation to do something is fine. But motivation can be fleeting while discipline is more reliable.

Gyms are full of motivated people the first week in January of each year. But over time, motivation begins to fade and some people quit working out. That is why it is more important to cultivate discipline.

To cultivate discipline means adding accountability, creating goals, and providing rewards for progress or penalties for failures. It is doing things that create less reliance on motivation. It is structure that creates results.

Jocko Willink led the most decorated Seal Team in Iraq. He noted that the highest performers on the team were those who had disciplined morning routines. They would wake up early to prepare for the day's mission while others slept. After his retirement, he started a consulting firm to bring his leadership knowledge to the business world. He presented the idea that discipline equaled freedom.

It was a concept that he believed helped to avoid micromanagement. He felt that when individuals were highly disciplined then they could be trusted to operate with little supervision. They would operate within standards agreed upon in advance. Everyone knew what everyone else would be doing and this discipline paradoxically created freedom. Seals under his command could respond quickly to a situation because they had a disciplined structure in place and didn't have to check with anyone before acting.

Most of this is mind over matter. If you want to be tougher, Jocko says be tougher. It is a decision.

Jocko said, "Accomplishing your goals isn't about motivation; it's about discipline."[18] Motivation is simply an influence. Discipline is training that molds. So while motivation is more like an external force, discipline is clearly internal and more within someone's control. Discipline is something that can be habitually ingrained. Jocko still wakes up at 4:30 every morning. He recommends making yourself do what you need to do over and over again. That is discipline.

Notes

1. Miyamoto Musashi, *The Five Rings, Miyamoto Musashi's Art of Strategy: The New Illustrated Edition of the Japanese Warrior Classic* (New York: Quarto Publishing Group, 2012).
2. Jeff Cooper, *Principles of Personal Defense* (Boulder, CO: Paladin Press, 2006).
3. Massad Ayoob, "New Info on Newhall," *American Handgunner* (1995), https://americanhandgunner.com/new-info-on-newhall/.
4. Thomas Aveni, "Officer-Involved Shootings," *The Police Policy Studies Council* (2003), http://www.theppsc.org/Staff_Views/Aveni/OIS.pdf.
5. Mike Gellatly, "Lucky for Him, Things Worked Out," *The Robesonian*, May 19, 2017.
6. K. S. Kendler et al., "The Genetic Epidemiology of Irrational Fears and Phobias in Men," *Archives of General Psychiatry* 5 (2001): 257–265.
7. John Taylor, "When Chamberlain and Russell Collided," *HQR News Weekend Edition Saturday* (2005), http://www.npr.org/templates/story/story.php?storyId=5036764.
8. Taylor Clark, "Do You Have Tiger Blood?" *Slate Magazine,* March 2011, http://www.slate.com/articles/arts/culturebox/2011/03/do_you_have_tiger_blood.html.
9. Ben Sherwood, "What It Takes to Survive a Crisis," *Newsweek*, January 23, 2009, http://www.newsweek.com/what-it-takes-survive-crisis-78207.
10. Lea Winerman, "Fighting Fire with Psychology," *American Psychological Association* 35 (2004): 28.
11. Glenn Llopis, "7 Ways Leaders Maintain Their Composure in Difficult Times," *Entrepreneur Magazine* (2014), https://www.entrepreneur.com/article/286581.
12. Jason McNeil, "Jhoon Rhee: Why Martial Arts Discipline May Be the Key to Happiness," *Black Belt Magazine*, May 2013, http://www.blackbeltmag.com/daily/martial-arts-philosophy/korean-martial-arts/jhoon-rhee-why-martial-arts-discipline-may-be-the-key-to-happiness/.
13. Your Warrior's Edge, "Warrior Quotes" (2017), http://yourwarriorsedge.com/warrior-quotes/.
14. *The Last Samurai*, directed by Edward Zwick, screenplay by John Logan.
15. Jeff Cooper, *To Ride, Shoot Straight, and Speak the Truth* (Boulder, CO: Paladin Press, 1988) p. 43.
16. Yasuka, "The Duel Between Sasaki Kojiro and Miyamoto Musashi," *KCP International Window on Japan*, January 26, 2015.
17. Peter Jacobs, "A Navy SEAL Commander Told Students to Make Their Beds in the Best Graduation Speech of 2014," *Business Insider*, April 16, 2015, http://www.businessinsider.com/mcraven-best-commencement-speech-university-texas-2015-4.
18. Richard Feloni, "Why This Retired Navy Seal Commander Has 3 Alarm Clocks and Wakes Up at 4:30 A.M.," *Business Insider*, Oct. 25, 2015, http://www.businessinsider.com/why-this-retired-navy-seal-has-three-alarm-clocks-2015-10.

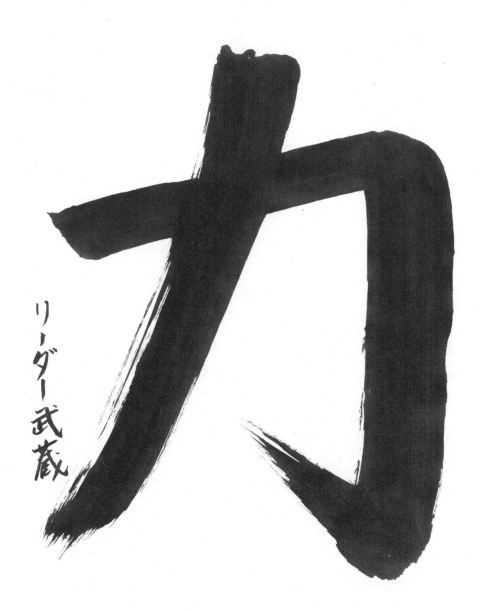

リーダー武蔵

PRINCIPLE SEVEN

POWER

POWER, OR FORCE, is mass multiplied by speed. Strength alone does not win fights. Power is the combination of speed and strength, which creates the necessary force to win. This explosive power wins fights.

Masutatsu Oyama, who was commonly referred to as Mas Oyama, was an influential master who founded Kyokushin karate. Though he was Korean, he spent most of his life in Japan. His name became synonymous with the power of martial arts.

In the 1950s, Oyama realized there were no good books he could recommend to foreigners that explained karate. He wrote a book called *What Is Karate*, first published in Japan. In the 1960s, the book was printed in English as *Mastering Karate*.[1] This work influenced many early martial artists, including myself, as it was one of the first exposures the West had to the power of martial arts.

Oyama was not only a full-contact karate champion. He was also known for fighting bulls barehanded. He battled 52 bulls in his lifetime. Three were reportedly killed instantly with one strike from Oyama, which earned him the nickname Godhand.

This was during the rise of Bruce Lee, who in 1964 appeared at the Long Beach International Karate Championships performing two-finger push-ups and a 1-inch punch that sent a larger man crashing to the floor. Bruce Lee was 5 foot 7 and weighed between 141 to 145 pounds. At one point in his life he was 165 pounds but reportedly felt the muscle mass at that size slowed him down, so he went back down to the low to mid-140s.[2]

There are some sources that recall Lee's training bags were customized to weigh 300 pounds.[3] Normal bags weigh from 70 to 150 pounds and are filled with light material. There are claims that Lee's were filled with metal and were heavier, not because he was showing off, but because he literally couldn't use the lighter bags. Normal bags were useless as he could kick one through the ceiling. It was his incredible speed that generated much of this power.

It was logical to conclude that Mas Oyama possessed great power, as he was physically a large man. But Bruce Lee captured even more attention with his martial arts power, which clearly emerged from speed, because he was much smaller.

It is often noted that while on the set of filming *The Green Hornet*, the footage had to be slowed down to capture Lee's movements. He was too fast for the film in that era. But there is even more to the power of both Oyama and Lee.

RESEARCH

In 2013, the journal *Cerebral Cortex* published a study titled, "Individual Differences in Expert Motor Coordination Associated with White Matter Microstructure in the Cerebellum."[4] In this academic study, the authors compared the behavior and brain structure of healthy control groups and karate black belts.

The researchers found that the black belts' motor coordination, experience, and age at which they began training were associated with individual differences in white brain matter integrity within the karate groups. This suggested training of neural responses in the brain that resulted in the ability to deliver blows like a 1-inch punch or to perform other tremendous feats of power. It was all about training the brain to coordinate the necessary elements and hardwiring them into the brain's structure. Biomechanical researchers recognize this power as coordination of the entire body to focus on a single explosive action in a process known as kinetic linking. Training changes the physical structure and function of the brain.

This process is seen in other sports as well and is at the cutting edge of training science.

Years of training this white matter enabled Oyama to break a bull's horn or even kill it with one strike, or allowed Bruce Lee to reportedly dislocate someone's shoulder with a slap.[5] Extraordinary coordination became ordinary to these martial artists.

Training enables the brain's neuroplasticity to literally rewire itself, which allows black belts to synchronize body movements and increase their power. So in a sense it is training for speed and coordination that produce the power. This training, speed, and coordination are continually developed by the fighter and are eventually hardwired into the neural cortex.

Mas Oyama notes in the introduction of his book that the source of karate's overwhelming effectiveness is an accumulation of ingenuity and wisdom over a long period of time in terms of the Oriental development of the combat arts. In terms of the individual, it is the result of constant training. The principles of combat haven't changed in thousands of years. Research simply confirms on the individual level that training in the application of these principles is quite effective.

APPLICATION

To exert power, a fighter must be able to strike an opponent harder, faster, and with the most efficient effort and avoid being hit effectively himself. This was the basis of Bruce Lee's power and the foundation of his work.

Lee felt a fighter should also have other qualities, such as the ability to move without telegraphing his movements. He believed that excellent coordination, which we've discussed in kinetic linking, was another quality along with balance and awareness. All of these qualities can be developed through training.

So strength and speed are synonymous with power, and this can be hardwired into the brain through training. A fighter can be strong, but if the fighter is slow and cannot hit a target then the fight will go to the swifter opponent. Power has many dimensions that transcend strength.

Many fighters can appreciate my personal experience of standing in a sweat-filled dojo for hours practicing the same punch over and over.

It is a universal experience. The tradition is timeless and it was Bruce Lee who noted its value, and credited with saying that he did not fear the man who has practiced 10,000 kicks once. He feared the man who has practiced one kick 10,000 times. More specifically, Lee referred to focusing wholeheartedly on a given task and having complete determination.[6]

Once such punch has one arm extended in front with the fist palm-side down. The other fist is cocked next to the chest with the palm side up. On the command of the sensei running the drill, the extended arm is pulled quickly backward as the cocked fist is punched forward. Both fists twist in synchronous fashion with the punching fist snapping just before contact. This punch exhibited explosive power and kinetic linking long before any scientific study was conducted on what created this power. But like Oyama opined, what we now know as kinetic linking was an accumulation of thousands of years of wisdom. Science now reveals that ancient fighters understood the physics of motion and how to maximize power. The power seemed mystical. But the power was simple physics.

POWER TO SCALE

The concept of speed and power applies on a larger scale as well. In World War II, Nazi Germany almost conquered all of Europe and North Africa by employing a technique referred to as the "blitzkrieg." This was lightning-fast war that was conducted with speed and concentrated power.[7]

Though it wasn't an official method, it delivered decisive, short battles that destabilized the other side before it could mobilize. The method did so by focusing overwhelming force on a small area of occupied territory to break through defenses. The problem was sustainability. Blitzkriegs worked but would run out of steam and outrun supply lines that fortified the attacking force. The pace of this power was short lived.

A fighter may also be able to overwhelm an opponent in the first round with this "blitz" of speed, power, and focused superiority. But the fighter had better finish the job, because if there is a second round the fighter with the most stamina will win. Boxing champion Floyd Mayweather Jr. is famous for picking apart his opponents in this manner. He is not a flashy fighter. He is patient and survives any blitz of power thrown at him. As a technical fighter he outlasts his opponent with his stamina, calmly surviving what comes his way.

This is what Germany experienced, as do many mixed martial arts fighters today. Sometimes it's not how much power you can dish out, but how much power you can absorb and keep coming back that counts. Germany was overextended and lacked a long-term strategy. They couldn't sustain the method they developed to employ rapid power. Speed counts. But it must be incorporated into a long-term strategy that is sustainable if the fight doesn't end quickly.

It was a sad evening at ringside one evening as I sat watching a series of fights with fellow members of the Boxing Commission. There was a group of several fighters who had the same trainer. They were in the red corner. They were all new and up against fighters who were essentially new as well, but had a different trainer. The latter group had been in the ring at least once. They were in the blue corner.

Things didn't look good when the first fighter in the red corner entered the ring and just stood there waiting on his opponent. The difference became apparent when the more experienced blue corner opponent entered the ring and started bouncing and warming up. The red corner fighter just stood there. He hardly moved.

Although the less-experienced red corner fighter didn't warm up and didn't look like he belonged in the ring, it was clear he wanted to win. He charged at the blue corner fighter swinging hard and often. The blue corner fighter simply dodged and weaved.

Soon the red corner fighter expended all his power. The swings slowed. It was then that the very first blows the blue corner fighter threw tagged the red corner fighter. The red corner fighter crumpled to the floor.

We observed that expending power quickly without discipline was not just one red fighter's choice. The same thing happened at least three times with his colleagues from the same gym and was the result of the team's training. Whether in war or in a ring, speed counts. But it is important to expend power efficiently. End the fight quickly. But understand the limits of your power so that speed doesn't overextend power.

CRUSH THE ENEMY

Chinese history is filled with examples of wars in which enemies were given mercy and allowed to live only to return and defeat those who had shown them leniency.

In his book *The 48 Laws of Power*, Robert Greene relates that in 1934, Communist leader Mao Tse-tung escaped the much larger army of Chiang Kai-shek. Chiang had decimated Mao's army. The original 75,000 men had dwindled to fewer than 10,000. Chiang determined that Mao was no longer a threat and gave up the pursuit. Mao was a devoted reader of Sun Tzu. A decade later his men recovered and destroyed Chiang, who had forgotten the warrior wisdom of destroying the enemy.[8]

Greene also reminds us of the first known instance of destroying the enemy. Egyptians pursuing Moses were completely destroyed by the Red Sea. The need to completely destroy the enemy is a fact as old as scripture.

Opponents do not wish you well. They wish to eliminate their opposition. It is a tenet of war that the opposition will act friendly only if defeated. Given time and the advantage, opponents will use power to defeat their enemies even if the opposition has shown mercy. This is why a necessity of fighting is to crush the enemy before the enemy crushes you.

Carl von Clausewitz was a scholar of war. He noted that after a war there was a time of negotiation and division of territory. If the victory was only partial, the parties could lose in negotiation what they had gained in battle.[9]

Von Clausewitz's solution was simple. Destroy the enemy to the point that they have no other option. They must be completely defeated, quickly and efficiently. That is the essence and goal of true power.

SPEED 101

Why is speed so important to power? How is it that someone as small as Bruce Lee can exert incredible power?

A quick physics lesson answers the question. Physics 101 demonstrates that the mass of an object increases with speed.[10] In other words, the faster an object moves, the more mass it attains. The higher the velocity of an object, like a fist or kick, the greater the impact.

Blame this concept on Einstein. Mass is simply potential energy. In the case of fighters we are talking about inertial mass. The faster an object travels, the greater the amount of energy that is exerted. We refer to this increase in energy as an increase in mass. Imagine throwing two rocks the exact same size. Whichever rock you throw the hardest will travel the fastest. The rock that travels the fastest will exert more striking power. It will hit harder. It doesn't hit harder because it's bigger than the other rock. It hits harder because it's moving faster. It's that simple. Now you know the secret behind Bruce Lee's punch.

So in our equation of power, let's say Superman and the Flash weigh nearly the same. They have similar mass. Though both fictional characters are fast, we assume the Flash is faster than Superman as speed is his primary superpower. The question then is, who would deliver the most powerful punch?

According to physics, the Flash would pack a more powerful punch. No one wants to get punched by Superman. But you really don't want to be punched by the Flash, who has physics on his side. That's how Bruce Lee did it and every martial artist should do it. Lee wasn't Superman or the Flash, he was simply fast and fast translates into power.

GENERATING POWER

Boxing is often more a punching contest than a power contest. While it is true that a brawler may rely on sheer strength in a fight, a brawler sacrifices accuracy, technique, and skill relying on strength alone to generate power. Experienced fighters generate more power through proper technique. Recall kinetic linking.

If a boxer has developed power through training, skill, and experience, then he has elevated the contest into much more than a punching match and tilts the odds of winning the fight to his favor.

Many athletes believe the development of power involves strength training through weight lifting. If their sport requires them to exert a pushing motion or action to move mass then this type of strength training will help. This is true with football, wrestling, or weight lifting.

But a punch or a kick is not a pushing motion. Striking is not an action designed to move mass. The goal of striking is to maximize impact. This requires execution of the velocity and mass equation using acceleration to exert force.

Many fighters don't know the difference. If a fighter doesn't understand the explosive kinetic energy of a snapping strike then the fighter's punches become exaggerated pushes like lifting weights.

Again, this is why Bruce Lee looked superhuman in the 1960s. He was really good but he wasn't superhuman. He was simply ahead of his time in terms of training, and he trained relentlessly. He understood kinetic linking, power, and acceleration. He understood speed and was fast. He was also a philosopher who could communicate many ancient concepts that had not been taught to fighters in the West for millennia. In fact, in the early days of his career, Lee was not very popular among Asians for teaching non-Asians.

Though there is nothing wrong with weight training, while other fighters were working on their strength, Lee was working on his speed. He lifted weights too, but he wanted long fast muscles and practiced coordinated movements that involved his whole body.

Relaxation when delivering a strike relieves the muscles of tension and allows the striking body part, such as a fist, to travel much faster without tension. Tension would slow down the strike. Then a brief contraction of muscles just before the strike combined with kinetic linking provides maximum impact. Kinetic linking is that snap, rotation, or pivot needed to incorporate the whole body into the strike. It involves the whole body starting with the feet, though the blow is delivered with the fist. This is why training with an experienced martial artist has value.

Muscle power alone cannot deliver a harder punch than your body weight in terms of force. The speed and technique with which that punch is delivered can increase the force. This is an important point regarding power. Speed translates into power.

Bruce Lee was not a big guy. But he could deliver devastating punches including his 1-inch punch. His speed is what amazed spectators. Speed along with technique can translate into incredible power. And there are mental aspects of power as well.

MENTAL POWER

The German philosopher Friedrich Nietzsche said that, "The value of a thing sometimes lies not in what one attains with it, but in what one pays for it—what it costs us."[11] The point here is whether or not to use power at all. It might help you to attain your goal, but at what cost?

If engaged in a fight, all the power at your disposal must be focused on the goal of winning the fight. The enemy should be crushed. But power can be used to avoid a fight as well. A decision must be made. Is using power to destroy the enemy worth the cost? In either case, the use of power must be disciplined. There is a time to use power and a time to withhold its use.

One of Sun Tzu's strategies of war was to make a small army seem large or vice versa.[12] Deception is a potent weapon when wielding power, and one way to manipulate its execution.

When walking alone on the street, it is better to appear strong, alert, and powerful especially if you are vulnerable. But if you are caring for a group of children, an air of power might scare them. The point is that power can be projected. Power is how others perceive it. Power is often perception in a mental sense.

One way to prevent a fight is to appear strong so that an attacker thinks it isn't worth the cost to start a fight. Cost works both ways. A bad guy may move on to an easier victim. Even the bad guys weigh the cost of a fight.

But if a fight is imminent, the fighter may wish to feign weakness to deceive the opponent regarding his strength. Like Sun Tzu, make the opponent think you are weak if you are actually strong but try to make the opponent believe you are strong if you are actually weaker. Again, power is perception. At least it is perceptual up to the point the power is actually executed. This is the interplay between the mental perception of power, how it is portrayed or displayed, and how it is actually delivered.

STRATEGIC POWER

Physical power comes from training to improve strength and endurance. But there are other sources of power as well.

Sun Tzu was referring to intellect or strategic thinking when he advised using deception as a tool. But strategic thinking is more than a tool. It is a source of power.

In the biblical story of David and Goliath, a small shepherd boy, David, volunteers to fight a giant, Goliath. But rather than putting on heavy armor, David chose to use only a slingshot. Without armor weighing him down he was able to move quickly. He stayed out of the reach of the much bigger Goliath. David defeated Goliath with shots from his slingshot, which is like shooting an unarmed opponent with a small caliber pistol today.

A fight isn't a test of only physical strength. David exerted his power through intellect and strategic thinking. This was a guerrilla-style tactic and has been used to exert power over a much larger opponent on many scales in many theaters of war.

We always refer to the story of David and Goliath as an example of the underdog defeating the champion. But in reality, Goliath never had a chance against David because David exhibited power through strategy.

EMOTIONAL POWER

There is an emotional source of power as well. Fighters call it having heart. In 1993, David Anspaugh directed a biographical sports film written by Angelo Pizzo on the life of Daniel "Rudy" Ruettiger, who played football at the University of Notre Dame despite overwhelming obstacles. The film, *Rudy*, is considered one of the top sports movies of all time.

Rudy dreamed of playing football for Notre Dame. He lacked the grades, talent, and money necessary to even attend the university. His physical stature and limited success on his high school football team limited him as well.

Rudy attended a nearby junior college to improve his grades and landed a minimum wage job as a groundskeeper at Notre Dame. Having little money, Rudy snuck into the groundskeeper's office to sleep.

After two years, Rudy was finally accepted to Notre Dame. He convinced the coach to accept him as a walk-on player who didn't have a sports scholarship. His spot was on the practice squad. The coach warned players that 35 scholarship players would not even be suiting up for games and the closest Rudy would get to playing was to get battered on the practice field.

Rudy never stopped driving himself 100 percent on the practice field. The coach noticed and promised to let him suit up for the last home game. The coach unexpectedly was replaced and the new coach didn't list Rudy on the play list for the last home game. Rudy decided to quit.

But the groundskeeper told Rudy he had played for Notre Dame and quit himself. He advised Rudy that he would regret it every day for the rest of his life if he quit. He reminded Rudy that he had nothing to prove to anyone but himself.

Upon Rudy's return to the team, the seniors all asked the coach to let Rudy take their place in the last game, laying their jerseys on the coach's desk. The coach relented and let Rudy suit up for the game against Georgia Tech.

With Notre Dame ahead 17–3, the coach sent all the seniors onto the field to play, except Rudy. The team scored a touchdown instead of running out the clock, as Rudy was a defensive player. With chants of "Rudy" in the background, the coach sent him in to play. Rudy sacked the Georgia Tech quarterback to the delight of the fans.

Rudy was then entered as an official member of the Notre Dame team and carried off the field on the shoulders of his teammates. Being carried off the field is a rare honor.

The scene of players laying their jerseys on the coach's desk was added for dramatic effect. But the point of the movie was the heart Rudy exerted throughout his time at Notre Dame. Despite the odds against him and his limited physical talent, he gave 100 percent every time he stepped on the playing field. Coaches wished they could take his heart and put it in the chest of bigger players. Rudy's heart or his emotional drive was the source of tremendous power and a good example of how far emotional strength can take someone. Athletes refer to this as leaving everything on the field as you put everything you had into the game.

SPIRITUAL POWER

There are more than just physical, intellectual, and emotional sources of power. There are spiritual sources as well. To Buddhists, the five spiritual qualities that become the five powers when exerted together are:[13]

1. Faith
2. Effort / Energy
3. Mindfulness
4. Concentration
5. Wisdom

The application is to have **faith** in happiness over material wealth but to exert **effort** or **energy** into doing positive things that pursue happiness as well. It is putting faith to action. The **mindfulness** component means to be present in the moment, as the past is behind us and worry of the future robs the present. **Concentration** is awareness and focus on specific tasks. The better we concentrate, the better we perform tasks. **Wisdom** provides the insight to understand these principles.

Power typically means physical energy. Sometimes it can mean authority. But this spiritual power is much deeper and is not just a tenet of Buddhism, but a foundation of every faith. It is a universal concept.

Because there is so much focus on the physical world in which we examine the use of physical power each day, most people have little awareness of spiritual power in another dimension. Spiritual power simply arises from another dimension and is invisible to those who only see the physical world. But it is a force.

The Christian scriptural approach invites followers to accept weakness in order to be strengthened. The apostle Paul said, "When I am weak, then I am strong" (2 Corinthians 12:10). This is the element of humility, which means accepting our limitations and relying on a higher power for strength. It is a value shared with other faiths such as Buddhism, in which humility is one of the 10 sacred qualities.[14]

The struggle is not with the physical world. It is a spiritual struggle. Have you noticed that to gain power in relationships you have to relinquish power? Spiritually, giving it up attains power. It is the law of reciprocity. It is even a law that science is beginning to understand and acknowledge.[15]

The law of reciprocity applies to nearly every culture. When someone gives you something you feel an obligation to give back. This is the concept of giving up power manifested spiritually. It is a paradox.

The Samurai followed Buddhist teachings in addition to Japan's native belief system of Shinto. They too understood this universal truth as servants relenting to a higher power. The Samurai were humble men who understood this spiritual aspect. They strove to attain enlightenment to achieve this spiritual power.

Musashi notes in his work, *The Book of Five Rings*, that the warrior lifestyle achieved levels of spirituality and referred to it as the path to enlightenment.[16] One of those warrior codes is to perceive that which cannot be seen. This spiritual component has traditionally been an important aspect of warrior culture throughout the ages. It is an ancient source of power that science is still struggling to understand. But a wise fighter can tap into this spiritual power that has been known to fighters throughout the ages.

POWER APPLICATION

While the superficial definition of power is moving an object from point A to point B quickly, or the ability to influence, we've seen there are many other types of power and sources of it as well. All have the similar concept of moving or influencing something else. It is simply the source from which the power is derived that differs.

In fighting, we exert a physical force. But the mental side of power must be ever present as well. In Shaolin teachings this concept was divided into two categories—Chan and Quan.[17] Chan refers to spiritual awareness and mastering perceptions of the mind. Quan refers to the physical. Shaolin Kung Fu masters understood that one encompasses the other.

This is how the concept of chi is associated with power. Chi is a force activated by mental awareness and focus that manifests itself physically. Chi is considered that which gives life. A biblical reference would be that which God breathed into man. It is a life force and the basis for much of Eastern medicine, such as acupuncture.

Practitioners of martial arts have strived to harness the power of chi for centuries. Ancient wisdom says that where the mind goes, chi will follow. It is this mental and physical integration of power that enables an elderly man in a Chinese park to toss much younger and stronger men around effortlessly. Practicing meditation, focus, and self-awareness are ways to develop chi.

Shaolin monks are living examples of this level of mastery. They focus mind, body, and emotions to harness incredible power. They understand the physical, mental, and spiritual components of power. They are in touch with their own mind, body, and soul. As a result of dedicating their lives to this level of mastery, they are able to exert a great deal of power.

Notice that these aspects of power transcend different fighting styles, physical size, or spiritual beliefs. This is because truth is truth regardless of its source. We are also finding that these truths of power are integrated into the laws of nature and are continually being discovered by science. To paraphrase American astronomer Robert Jastrow, when scientists have scaled the highest mountain of ignorance, as they pull themselves over the final rock, they will be greeted by a band of theologians who have been sitting there for centuries. The Samurai understood all the sources of power. Sun Tzu understood all the sources of power. We are still learning and discovering them ourselves.

Power must be cultivated and refined. Ultimately, its connection to speed must also be realized. It also must be understood as the result of many sources. It is then that true power is achieved.

Notes

1. Mas Oyama, *Mastering Karate* (New York: Grosset & Dunlap, 2017).
2. Chris Trevino, "Bruce Lee Put US Martial Arts on the Grand State in Long Beach 50 Years Ago," *Press-Telegram*, August 1, 2014, http://www.presstelegram.com/sports/20140801/bruce-lee-put-us-martial-arts-on-the-grand-stage-in-long-beach-50-years-ago.
3. East Meets West International, "Bruce Lee Heavy Bag Training," n.d., http://eastmeetswest.com/bruce-lee-heavy-bag-training/.
4. R. E. Roberts et al., "Individual Differences in Expert Motor Coordination Associated with White Matter Microstructure in the Cerebellum," *Cerebral Cortex* 23 (2013): 2282–2292.
5. M. Uyehara, *Bruce Lee: The Incomparable Fighter* (Chicago: Black Belt Communications, 1988), 32.
6. John Little, *The Warrior Within: The Philosophies of Bruce Lee* (London: Chartwell Books, 2016), 161.

7. C. Trueman, "Blitzkrieg," *The History Learning Site,* August 16, 2016, http://www.historylearningsite.co.uk/world-war-two/world-war-two-and-eastern-europe/blitzkrieg/.

8. Robert Greene, *The 48 Laws of Power* (New York: Penguin Books, 1998), 111–113.

9. Carl von Clausewitz, *On War* (New York: Barnes & Noble, 2004).

10. Sten Odenwald, "Special and General Relativity Questions and Answers," *NASA Astronomy Café,* n.d., https://einstein.stanford.edu/content/relativity/q389.html.

11. Michael Jackson, *The Work of Art: Rethinking the Elementary Forms of Religious Life* (New York: Columbia University Press, 2016), 162.

12. Sun Tzu, *The Art of War and Other Classics of Eastern Thought* (New York: Barnes & Noble, 2013).

13. Barbara O'Brien, "The Five Powers," *ThoughtCo* (2017), https://www.thoughtco.com/the-powers-of-buddhism-449707.

14. Chen Yu-Hsi, "The Buddhist Perception of Humility," *International Network on Personal Meaning,* n.d., http://www.meaning.ca/archives/archive/art_buddhist-humility_C_Yu_Hsi.htm.

15. David Jensen, "The Law of Reciprocity," *Science,* February 15, 2013, http://www.sciencemag.org/careers/2013/02/law-reciprocity.

16. Miyamoto Musashi, *The Five Rings, Miyamoto Musashi's Art of Strategy: The New Illustrated Edition of the Japanese Warrior Classic* (New York: Quarto Publishing Group, 2012).

17. Craig Sands, "The Importance of Training the Mind in Wing Chun," *Wing Chun Journey,* https://wcjourney.wordpress.com/the-journey/the-importance-of-training-the-mind-in-wing-chun/.

集中

リーダー 武蔵

FOCUS

TAKEDA SHINGEN was a Japanese feudal lord feared for his military tactics. He rose to power as a young warrior and sought to control the nearby Shinano province. As many as four well-known warlords became aware of his desire and decided to quickly defeat the young Shingen before he could become too powerful.[1]

These warlords amassed a 12,000-man army to face Takeda Shingen's 3,000. As the warlords took up positions along the border, Shingen's forces unexpectedly attacked in a precise location killing 3,000 and losing only 500 of their own. Though the warlords were prepared and had over-whelming power, Takeda Shingen focused his strength, pushing into the province while the warlords were still confused. Shingen's skillful focus, combined with the element of surprise, outweighed his opponent's power and preparation.

This is the paradox of the ancient principles of winning fights. All the principles are interrelated and the fighter who executes them best wins. You begin to see how these principles converge.

Discipline, for example, directs a fighter to possess a controlled calmness during a fight. But it is the principle of focus that gives discipline clarity. All principles of fighting are interconnected; and each principle encompasses the others. Each principle complements or counters another.

But it is focus that brings their effectiveness together so that each can be applied in an efficient manner.

MANAGING FOCUS

Focus has a broad sense and a narrow sense. From the broader perspective, let's consider that everyone has the same amount of time. For example, Einstein, Reagan, and Churchill all had 24 hours in a day. They got great things accomplished through focus, not time.

How about the epic task of writing a novel? With only a few dozen novels, Stephen King is considered a prolific author. Yet he has nothing on Isaac Asimov, who published more than 460 books in all but one of the ten major categories of the Dewey Decimal System. All these great thinkers, leaders, and authors had the same amount of time but each controlled their focus better than the average person.

What about physical training to be great? All fighters have the same amount of time in a day to train. Every athlete, from Muhammad Ali to Bruce Lee, each chooses how to focus his or her time.

The question becomes, How do great minds, leaders, innovators, writers, or fighters find the time to become great and accomplish all that they do? It can't be said enough that the difference is they manage their focus rather than their time. Focus concentrates the necessary components to win in terms of managing thought, energy, and time.

Managing the use of energy is the key to accomplishing great things in a broad sense. This is sometimes called working smart rather than working hard. To accomplish complex or huge tasks requires the ability to maximize the available time rather than adding hours to the day.

NARROW FOCUS

This narrow focus is all about concentrating strength. Ancient practitioners developed effective arts based on the application of physics and accomplished seemingly impossible feats. While it is clear that larger fighters have greater potential energy, ancient masters understood there were ways to express, redirect, or otherwise focus energy to any practitioner's advantage regardless of size. They understood physics and maximized energy by focusing these physical laws.

For example, a larger fighter might deliver his potential energy in an inefficient manner by swinging wildly with the energy of his muscular arm, while the smaller fighter, who is working smarter not harder, focuses a punch onto a relatively small area with concentrated force delivered by driving a larger percentage of his potential energy from his legs, hips, and through to his arm then fist in a snapping focused manner. This is kinetic linking as previously discussed in Principle Seven: Power.

The larger fighter used his arm. The smaller smarter fighter used his whole body and focused the point of impact, thus maximizing the force. The fighter who focuses energy best gets more done. Just like great thinkers and leaders, a fighter accomplishes more by simply managing focus.

I can remember standing in line with other young martial artists as a teenager. Anyone who has trained knows the drill. On command we stepped and punched, stepped and punched, stepped and punched. This exercise literally went on for hours. We thought its purpose was to weed out those who weren't willing to muster the discipline to perform a repetitious skill over and over. But it was training the focus of punches to perfection so that it was embedded in muscle memory forever. Science now understands the value in this time-honored training.

Whether on the broad or narrow level, focus is about managing energy. There are also mental aspects of focusing to win fights, such as eliminating distractions that would interfere with focusing energy.

When practicing, a martial artist focuses 100 percent on doing martial arts. Just like a pianist should be 100 percent focused when playing or a writer should be focused totally on writing when writing.

When fighting, there can be no distractions. On the macro level, the focus is on the fight. On the micro level, it is on concentrating energy.

BALANCED FOCUS

The broad focus should be on the overall fight and not just elements of the attack. If there is too much focus on a specific attack then a counter attack might be missed. Concentrating on the fighter rather than the specifics of the fight is a difficult skill to master.

Intense focus on an opponent's punches will cause the fighter to lose sight of the opponent's kicks, for example. Obsession with the right hand that you keep blocking will cause you to miss seeing the left hand that knocks you out. A balanced view of the fighter and not simply the fight is difficult to achieve.

So it's more about not focusing on the wrong thing. If a fighter focuses on a weapon or punch to such a degree he doesn't see the weapon in the other hand or a kick coming from another direction then he will be defeated.

It's like a magician's sleight of hand. You concentrate so hard you limit the processing capacity of the parietal cortex in the brain so as not to pay attention to different information. While concentrating on the right hand you don't see what the left is doing. Focus is all about balancing awareness.

On the street you can execute a perfect takedown of an opponent then apply the perfect arm bar on one of his arms—just as you learned in class. But if you didn't balance your focus and failed to notice the knife he pulled out of his pocket with the other arm you would encounter something you did not practice in class. While your legs and both arms are tied up in the perfect arm bar, your lack of balanced awareness would result in the opponent stabbing you with his other arm while you lay on your back. Focus should not put blinders on your fight; it should center your fight.

Genki desu ka?[2] This is Japanese for "How are you?" Notice the *ki* in the first word. It is the same *ki* we use to refer to energy in martial arts. You will sometimes see it written as *chi* or *gi* in Chinese. Literally translated it means, "Is your energy centered?"

Two Japanese words, *ki* and *ai*, mean "energy" and "join." Together, they form the word *kiai*, which is shouted when performing martial arts. So a *kiai* is not simply screaming or yelling, but delivers stored energy in a focused, explosive fashion. Balanced focus centers the fight in attempts to eliminate blind spots.

MUSHIN

Another concept regarding focus is *mushin*. This is the shortened version of *mushin no shin*, which means "the mind without mind."[3] The concept isn't about emptying the mind and thinking about nothing as much as ridding the mind of distractions. It is not something the ancients believed could be understood by intellect alone but instead must be experienced. It is a mind that is fully awake but clear of distracting thoughts or emotions.

It is the ability to stay calm, taking in your opponent's actions dispassionately. The closest English translation for the concept of mushin is "disinterested." This is not the same as "uninterested," but rather impartial, flexible, and unbiased. In Eastern thought, the concept is to have a still center. It is being calm without outside influences affecting this center.

Mushin is about being fully aware and focused on the moment: a state of mental clarity and perception not distracted by emotion or fixed thought. In a state of mushin the warrior is intensely aware and focused on the moment but detached at the same time. Movements are intuitive and not guided by conscious thought. It is a beautiful state once the concept is understood, though again, being fully present but fully detached at the same time is difficult to describe.

Takuan Soho was a Zen Buddhist monk and founder of one of the most famous Japanese sword schools in the sixteenth century.[4] He was a contemporary and friend to the great warrior Miyamoto Musashi. Takuan said that the proper focus of the mind was that it should be continuously flowing. It should not stop anywhere, which would be injurious to the mind's well-being. This is a concept he referred to as the unfettered mind. It was an idea the monk felt applied to all areas of life.

The mind should be like water flowing freely. It shouldn't get stuck in one spot like water that has frozen. Bruce Lee said the fighter must be shapeless and formless, like water. He said that when water is poured into a cup, it becomes the cup. When water is poured into a bottle, it becomes the bottle. When water is poured into a teapot, it becomes the teapot. Water can drip according to Lee. It can also crash. Bruce Lee said the fighter should become water.[5] His original quote appeared on the TV series *Longstreet* in 1971 when Bruce Lee played the part of a martial arts instructor.

Although the concept of mushin seems paradoxical to focus, it is actually symbiotic. In a strategic sense, the mind should be open, flowing, and not distracted by extraneous thought in a fight, particularly emotions such as fear or specific actions. Takuan described this in terms of facing a single tree. If you look at a single leaf, you will miss all the others. It is an important clarity of focus that must be understood. Buddhist monks attempt to perfect this mind-set. This isn't the typical Western view of focus, which we correlate to simply concentration. Focus is removing distractions and allowing the mind to flow like water around the thoughts requiring full attention at the moment.

PHYSICAL FOCUS

In addition to a focused mind, there is tactical focus to consider as well. Tactical focus refers to the concept that once an action is committed then all the energy to execute the action must converge at the precise point requiring the action. This is a merging of all the necessary energy into one point. It is a major component of striking through a target rather than simply striking at it. This is the physical sense of focus. Striking through the target at a precise point is the most efficient manner to focus energy.

Focused basketball players make higher percentages of their free throws than unfocused players. Keeping your eye on the goal despite distractions is essential. It requires training to attain this focus by training with distractions, consequences, and stress to acclimate performance under realistic conditions. It was a skill practiced by the ancient masters who were able to use focus in both its broad and narrow sense to accomplish their goal. This enables the fighter to not only access the conscious cerebral cortex where general thoughts are managed but the unconscious cerebellum portion of the brain, which is needed for managing complex intricate movements. Things are more hard-wired in the cerebellum.

Recall that Bruce Lee referred to early training in martial arts as a punch was just a punch and a kick just a kick. But with more training a punch or kick became a series of thoughts and actions. Distance, range, timing, and strike points were things a fighter thought about while practicing punches and kicks. But when the fighter mastered these movements over time, a punch then became just a punch, and a kick, just a kick. It became simple again.[6] Focus is more than concentrating. Focus is hard-wiring movements into the brain so that concentration is on the small things and the whole picture is effortless. Many movements can then be accomplished simultaneously.

In the movie *The Patriot*,[7] Mel Gibson's character teaches a small boy how to shoot. The boy is told to aim small, miss small. It is a fundamental technique of aiming a shot by aiming at the smallest point of the target as possible—like aiming at a coat button on an enemy rather than the enemy in general. Aim at something the size of a quarter rather than at the target as a whole. The shooter may miss the small object but will still hit the target. The concept is to aim in a focused manner rather than shooting aimlessly. (As a side note, you should also practice not moving the gun as well, or focusing your aim means nothing.)

LIFE FOCUS

Life should have the same focus. Ephesians 5:17 says, "Don't act thoughtlessly, but understand what the Lord wants you to do." These words, written by the apostle Paul, urge one to not live carelessly but to make certain there is focus in accomplishing God's mission. It is a tenet of many religions. Buddhists practice meditation that clears the mind and concentrates their focus, making the meditator more fully aware. Focus arises from these sources. Focus bridges spiritual and physical aims.

Focusing on a problem by worrying aimlessly about it will not solve the problem. It will only magnify it. Focusing on solutions is a life lesson of many faiths. Even the *Star Wars* character Qui-gonn Jinn understands this. He advised Anakin to "always remember, your focus determines your reality."[8]

Fighting, shooting, and living life should all be done with focus. Laser-beam focus concentrates power on one spot. In a fight, focus should be on a single point for maximum impact. In life, we should concentrate on one thing at a time. Confucius said, "He who chases two rabbits catches none."[9]

Focus will allow you to achieve goals more quickly, and you will be more productive. Choose one thing to focus on at a time. Eliminate distractions, which are the enemy of focus. Practice with distractions lessens the impact of distractions during real performance.

Calm the mind of internal distractions as well. Internal talk or extraneous thoughts prevent proper focus on a task. Declutter both the surrounding environment and the mind. Understanding goals and simplifying life also aid focus.

Most people do not understand the capacity of energy they can command if they simply focus everything on a single point. Breaking a board, writing a book, or achieving any goal is accomplished through these same methods. Managing focus, not time, is the secret.

Have you watched a martial artist who breaks bricks? He stands before them, clears his mind, declutters thoughts and distractions while understanding his goal of breaking through the mass. His task is simple and his focus is sharp. Breaking bricks or sending a man to the moon are both achieved through focus.

In his 1998 book, *Creating Affluence: The A to Z Steps to a Richer Life*, Deepak Chopra expresses the idea that intention (goals) transforms while attention (focus) creates.[10] So if we select a single task and assemble complete focus on the task until it is complete, the results are amazing. It sounds simple, but much of life is devoid of this type of single-minded focus.

Basketball players and other athletes talk about being in the zone. The past and the present do not matter. They are totally immersed in their current task and time vanishes. It is the state of mind that Samurai attempted to achieve on the battlefield, as it is at this moment the mind and body are most effective.

Best-selling author Sebastian Junger[11] is also a documentary filmmaker. Junger and Tim Hetherington co-directed *Restrepo*, a 2010 documentary that was nominated for an Academy Award. The film chronicled a year with a platoon of U.S. soldiers deployed to the Korengal Valley in Afghanistan.

Junger related in numerous interviews that the Special Forces soldiers behaved differently than some of the other soldiers. Immediately upon hearing an attack was imminent they became very calm.[12] More specifically, he said their cortisol levels would drop. The reason was that the unknown was stressful for them, but knowing they were about to be attacked had a calming effect because they could then focus on a plan of action.

They filled sandbags, prepared weapons, and stockpiled ammunition. This focus gave them control over their environment, even in the face of danger. They immersed themselves in a task and were in the zone.

There are only three possible reactions to everything you face:

1. Accept it.
2. Change it.
3. Leave it.

Tension is not caused by making a decision. People sit around wishing they had changed something. They wonder what should they do. They may let worry linger, not accepting something if they can't change it. Once a decision is made then the stress is gone and the focus can begin on fulfilling the decision. Decide, and then focus on the decision. Indecision is what causes stress.

Special operators in war understand this and it is the reason they aren't worried about an attack. They know it's coming. They accept it. They then focus their plan.

The vast majority of a person's effort is wasted because of a lack of focus. Energy should be concentrated on whether an action is going to put you closer to your goal. Even thoughts should be evaluated. Why are you having the thought and is it productive? Focus everything. Again, efficiency is not managing time, it is managing focus.

Spiritual teacher Eckhart Tolle is the author of several books. In *The Power of Now* he says that enlightenment is the space between your thoughts.[13] This space emanates peace not of this world according to Tolle. Focusing on the present is a feature of his message. When met with difficulty the old phrase, "This too shall pass" is a reality check for our mind to focus on what is important.

To win fights, focus the mind on principles. Then focus the body on action as good technique follows principles. Direct all your energy on one focal point to drive through the goal whether it is a mental goal or a physical opponent. Focus and drive through it.

Focus can be achieved through realistic practice. But understand it has many facets, both spiritual and physical. You must access the conscious and the unconscious. Manage focus and you manage time, because focused fighters win.

NOTES

1. Phillip Duncan, "Takeda Shingen: Legendary Strategist and the Tiger of Kai," *Hubpages, History of Asia*, May 16, 2012, https://hubpages.com/education /Takeda-Shingen-Legendary-Strategist-and-the-Tiger-of-Kai.
2. Simon Ager, "Useful Japanese Phrases," *Omniglot: The Online Encyclopedia of Writing Systems and Languages* (2017), http://www.omniglot.com/language /phrases/japanese.php.
3. Christopher Caile, "Mushin: The State of Mind," Fightingarts.com, http://www .fightingarts.com/reading/article.php?id=62.

4. Takuan Soho, *The Unfettered Mind* (n.d.), http://www.alexandrosmarinos.com/TheUnfetteredMind.pdf.

5. *Longstreet* TV series, "The Way of the Intercepting Fist," directed by Don McDougall, written by Stirling Siliphant. Paramount TV: September 16, 1971.

6. Tony Fryer, "The Science Behind Your Free Throws," *USA Basketball*, January 28, 2010, https://www.usab.com/youth/news/2010/01/the-science-behind-your-free-throws.aspx; Elizabeth Svoboda, "How to Avoid Choking under Pressure," *Scientific American*, February 2009.

7. *The Patriot*, directed by Roland Emmerich, screenplay by Robert Rodat (2000).

8. *Star Wars: The Phantom Menace*, directed and written by George Lucas (1999).

9. David Roads, "Person Who Chases Two Rabbits Catches Neither," *Philosiblog*, October 31, 2013, http://philosiblog.com/2013/10/31/person-who-chases-two-rabbits-catches-neither/.

10. Deepak Chopra, *Creating Affluence: The A to Z Steps to a Richer Life* (Novato, CA: New World Library, 1998).

11. Sebastian Junger, *The Perfect Storm* (New York: Harper Perennial, 2006).

12. Sebastian Junger, "Sebastian Junger on the Thrill and Hell of 'War' Excerpt," *HQR News Special Series*, May 11, 2010, http://www.npr.org/2010/05/11/126676276/sebastian-junger-on-the-thrill-and-hell-of-war.

13. Eckhart Tolle, *The Power of Now: A Guide to Spiritual Enlightenment* (London: Yellow Kite, 2001).

激烈

リーダー 武蔵

FIERCENESS

MAHATMA GANDHI said that if the only options were cowardice and violence, he would advise violence.[1] It is a deep concept from such a peaceful man. Gandhi was a master of nonviolence but understood the need for violence to defend the innocent or those who were oppressed.

A warrior may choose pacifism. But a pacifist who is a coward is condemned to pacifism with no other choice and no other option. Just because someone has the potential for violence, has the means to produce violence, and is a warrior willing to commit violent acts, doesn't mean a warrior is inherently violent. But it provides the warrior with options. To really win fights, this violence must be taken to an extreme to ensure victory once a violent path is chosen as a solution.

Being fierce is displaying ferocious aggressiveness. The term "ferocious" is often used to describe the lion, which is considered to be the "king of the jungle." "Ferocious" means extremely violent and aggressive and sometimes intensely destructive. Being ferocious is to be brutal, vicious, and even barbarous or merciless in action.

In Lt. Col. Jeff Cooper's work on gun fighting, he included the principles of aggressiveness and ruthlessness as necessary for effective self-defense, which are essentially subsets of the principle of fierceness. Ferocity encompasses these fierce ancient concepts of the brutality needed to win battles. It is simply a fact of war, or other life and death situations: to win a fight one must be extremely violent. The most violent fighter will typically win because a fighter must be vicious when the fighting begins.

Many police departments rejected these principles that Cooper suggested in his seminars as they are bound by strict rules of engagement when confronting violence. Ruthlessness and aggression did not fit with their mission as primarily peacekeepers. Long guns were placed in the trunk of the patrol car out of sight. Police cars were even painted with less aggressive colors.[2] This is the position of many police administrations as guardians in a civil society.

Fierceness is simply a broader term that can be scaled and hopefully balances this view that the words "aggressiveness" and "ruthlessness" are too strong. Ferocity provides the image of a lion protecting the pride by means of his ferocious presence demonstrated by his roar, while ruthless aggression may seem a callous term that provokes negative images. The underlying principle is the same. The term simply provides clarity.

The point of ferocity is that overwhelming violence is necessary to win a fight. Explosive, aggressive, and even cold-hearted ruthless action is at the core of winning violent confrontations. It is this brutal reality that peace-loving people abhor and with good reason. Nevertheless, winning a fight means to be relentless in pursuit of winning it. While police or other guardians of peace may need to scale down their expression of violence, it must be understood that this doesn't change the underlying principle. The more violent fighter will generally win, as it is simply the physics of fighting.

Rationally and legally, no more force should be utilized than is necessary to neutralize a threat.[3] This is scaling the force of the ferocity. But the amount of necessary force can be a nebulous thing in the heat of battle. Fortunately, ferocity is mutually exclusive of the amount of force in many ways. Ferocity itself is simply an expression of an explosive and aggressive response to an attack without specifically accounting for force. Each individual must decide how to scale that force depending on a given situation. A fierce fighter will win. How much fierceness is necessary depends on the situation. But fundamentally, fierceness wins, as it can make up for other deficiencies such as size.

A small bird can ferociously defend her nest against larger animals causing a stronger animal to flee in fear. Clearly, the larger animal possessed the required force and power to defeat a small bird. But the ferocity of the small bird can overcome greater force. This is the paradox of ferocity. Focused, explosive aggression can allow for less force to be applied to neutralize a situation. The roar of a ferocious lion will keep enemies at bay, as they understand the potential strength behind the aggressive action. The expression of aggression must be present if actual physical force is to be lowered, as opponents respect strength over weakness.

You can stop delivering force once the attack is neutralized. But up until that point the fighter must be overwhelmingly explosive to win and get the fight to the point it can be neutralized. If the fighter is aggressive he will reach that point more quickly. In this sense, being a fierce fighter can actually bring an end to violence more quickly. This is the reward of aggression.

Fighting with ferocity may seem cruel. But just as an attacker must be met with similar force to stop the attack, the fierce mind-set must be similar as well in order to prevent delay in counterattacking or surviving. The attacker is callus and shows no compassion or humanity, as evidenced by an attack on an innocent person. A severe brutal response is the most successful response to an unfeeling attacker. A humane response may not defeat an inhuman attack if it doesn't possess its own element of brutality.

Savage fierceness is a quality of being ferocious. Ferocity is being bold, wild, and expressing a bit of surprise as well. Ferocity implies being more intense than expected. Developing confidence is a way to foster this principle. Confidence along with turning fear into anger will result in fierceness.

BUDO

There are many paradoxes found in the history of the principles presented here. Ferocity is one of them, as it seems to conflict with the humble nature of ancient monks who perfected these principles. It is paradoxical that such peaceful men could become so fierce during battle. But it is more paradoxical in the Western view.

The Japanese term *budo*, which is translated as "martial art," is a prime example of this contrast. Westerners noted the vigor with which Asian practitioners approached budo or martial arts. The Western concept of budo was the way of the warrior, the martial way or warlike.

The Eastern concept is much different, however. The character for *bu* is made up of other characters meaning "arms of war" or "violence" and "to stop" or "bring to an end." The character for *do* means "the way."[4]

A more accurate translation might be to stop violence or to bring about peace. It is the art of the peacemaker in this view, though in the Western view it is the art of war. Warfare and strength are necessary to bring about peace. This principle is as ancient as time itself.

Peace is the ultimate goal in the Eastern view. Violence is an unfortunate necessity that is sometimes required to win peace. Violence results when other ways of solving a problem fail.

Ronald Reagan popularized the phrase "peace through strength" during the cold war.[5] Roman Emperor Hadrian used the phrase as early as the first century. During the fourth century, Latin author Publius Flavius Vegetius Renatus wrote that those who want peace must prepare for war (*"Si vis pacem, para bellum"*). George Washington, Abraham Lincoln, and Margaret Thatcher all paraphrased this concept during speeches. Will Rogers observed that he had never seen anyone insult the world heavyweight champion, Jack Dempsey.[6] Peace through strength is a timeless concept.

On August 6, 1945, the American bomber *Enola Gay* dropped a five-ton bomb over Hiroshima, Japan.[7] It was a massively destructive act. But in many ways it saved lives, as advisers had warned President Harry S. Truman that invading the Japanese mainland would result in horrific American casualties. The action quickly resulted in peace, and this aggressive action may have saved lives.

The best way to stop aggressive dictators, enemies, or terrorists is if they know you have the means, and the will to use those means, to stop them at all costs. The same is true on a personal level. Criminals interviewed in prison have repeatedly listed fear of the victim as the number one deterrent to crime.[8] Criminals say they do not fear laws, police, alarms, dogs, or other methods as much as they fear a victim who is armed or has the ability to harm them.

Winston Churchill once said that an appeaser is one who feeds a crocodile hoping it will eat him last.[9] An attacker will take advantage of any perceived weakness, as attacking weakness is a common tactic of winning a fight. This is why appeasement is seldom an option. Compliance with an aggressor is a calculated risk that puts the attacker in control. When and how much a victim complies is an individual decision, depending on the situation. But once an opportunity presents itself, crushing the enemy is the best option once physical confrontation is the decided course of action. Sun Tzu wrote that the fighter who knows when to fight and when not to fight will be victorious.[10] But once the fight has begun the enemy should be crushed.

MMA

As noted previously, our team once prepared a fellow black belt for a cage fight. It was to be his first time competing in a full contact event. Technically, he was the very best. He was great on his feet. He was a perfect technician on the ground. He was fit, trained incessantly, and was favored to win. However, he lost his first fight. The reason was clear and fits with the concept of fierceness as well.

The black belt was a nice guy. While this is a great quality, he didn't have what fighters refer to as a mental switch. You can be a nice guy outside the ring or away from a fight. But once you enter the ring or once a fight begins that switch must be flipped in the fighter's mind. The fighter may be the nicest guy in the world. But when the fight begins he must be the meanest. He must be the nastiest. He must be the most aggressive and brutal. He simply must be ferocious. He cannot be that nice guy in the fight.

Our guy never flipped the switch. He therefore was holding back a bit by not being fierce. His ferocity did not come through and it cost him the fight.

VIOLENCE

Don't imagine that you can reason with an attacker. Many times they have less to lose than you do. Therefore, if you cannot escape or if it is sport fighting that is planned or even an unavoidable full-scale war, the way to end the fight is to be more ferocious and more violent than the opposition.

Experts on violence have noted that the goal of a criminal is to control his victim.[11] Everything he says and does is intended to terrify, intimidate, and control. In many cases, the more control the criminal is given the less likely the victim will escape.[12] Time works against the victim of violence and favors the criminal aggressor. This is why there must be a swift reaction to escape, or to violently react with greater ferocity if escape is not an option. To win requires being more savage than the attacker and is the only way to take back control.

The movie franchise *John Wick* is a prime example of ruthless brutality overwhelming opponents.[13] John Wick, played by Keanu Reeves, is an antihero. Reeves received real-world firearms training from world champion shooter Taran Butler, who runs Taran Tactical Innovations. The shooting style embodies fierce principles of fighting and has been referred to as "gun fu."

The Wick character is a stoic but ruthless hit man feared by other hit men because he is committed, focused, and disciplined. He is also very brutal and is referred to as the Baba Yaga or bogeyman. The Russian mobsters in the film describe him as the man you send to kill the bogeyman.

The Baba Yaga is a supernatural being from Slavic folklore.[14] Often depicted as an old witch, she never bothers anyone if not provoked and can be either a benefactor or a villain. The Baba Yaga has few morals and in some folklore is considered to be the devil's grandmother. Calling John Wick the Baba Yaga puts the character into the Russian mobster culture and epitomizes his complex nature along with his power.

John Wick's back is tattooed with the Latin words, *Fortis Fortuna Adiuvio*.[15] Literal translations attribute this as "Fortune Favors the Bold," which is the motto of the Third Marine Regiment based in Hawaii where the actor has roots. But the Third Marine Regiment motto is actually *Fortes Fortuna Juvat* (sometimes seen as *iuvat*). *Fortis* is actually the plural form of a noun meaning "individual strength." Fortuna is the Roman goddess of luck. *Adiuvio* is to save or help. So a more accurate translation is, "It is only the Strong that Fortuna comes to save" or "Fortune favors the strong." Is this the opposite of the biblical notion that the meek shall inherit the earth? Actually, there are parallels rather than oppositions.[16] You might be surprised to learn the true meaning of meekness that is valued by the world's religions.

There is a misconception that meek means to be passive or weak. The Greek New Testament word is *praus* and does not suggest weakness.[17] It means mild disposition or gentleness of spirit. It involves self-control and the scriptural application is one who is not easily provoked. *Praus* calls to mind a calm captain of a ship, who remains stoic in the midst of a storm. It is strength under control. The Greeks utilized the term to describe a wild horse that is tamed. In the biblical sense, being meek defines a person who focuses strength in a controlled fashion in God's service.

These parallels have little to do with John Wick, who certainly doesn't exhibit typical hero qualities and is actually an antihero. However, the character John Wick does exhibit the controlled calm nature of someone with focus who is able to unleash unparalleled raw brutality to win.

FEROCIOUS WARRIORS

Genghis Khan was born around 1162.[18] He created the Mongol Empire, which was one of the largest empires in the world. He organized a large army and was feared for his merciless brutality. Khan and his Mongol army destroyed city after city if they opposed him. They swept through fortifications slaughtering everything in sight. Even small domestic animals were killed. Any survivors were marched in front of the army as shields as they attacked the next fortification.

Khan would send out an order for a city to surrender or die. If they did not surrender he would massacre the entire populace. Author Steven Pinker notes in his book, *The Better Angels of Our Nature*,[19] that Khan may have wiped out as many as 40 million people. Even a small Mongol occupying force could subdue a much larger populace as people feared that if they overpowered the smaller Mongol army a larger one would exact retribution.

For all his ruthless methods, goods, information, medicine, and technology traveled freely under Khan's rule. He abolished torture and class systems. He promoted soldiers based on their ability rather than social class. While the world feared Khan, his men were loyal to him.

In the fourteenth century, the Mings overthrew the Mongol-led Yuan dynasty. To solidify their new Ming dynasty, they rounded up all Mongol males. Any who were taller than a wagon wheel were killed immediately. Any male children shorter than a wagon wheel were castrated and girls were taken as concubines. The policy was therefore to kill the men, castrate the boys, and take the women.[20] Ruthless brutality and swift action has developed some of the greatest military commanders throughout history.

Around 335 BCE, Alexander the Great became ruler of Macedonia at twenty years of age.[21] Taking advantage of his young age and recent crowning, the citizens of Thebes revolted. They massacred the occupants of a Macedonian garrison and declared their independence.

Alexander was yet to be called great. He quickly marched into Thebes and punished the insurgents mercilessly. His forces burned the city and any survivors were sold as slaves. He carried out this attack before the citizens realized what had happened. His swift and brutal action set the stage for developing one of the largest empires in history.

Beyond individual fighters renowned for their brutality as the key to their success, the most successful martial arts have a fierce ruthlessness at the center of their effectiveness as well. Specifically, hand-to-hand combat arts are designed not to break boards but people.

FEROCIOUS METHODS

Krav maga is one example of an effective hand-to-hand combat system. Developed by the Israel Defense Forces,[22] it consists of a wide combination of techniques derived from many martial arts, utilizing those that are effective in real fights. Its focus is to end a fight quickly. The method targets vulnerable body areas such as the eyes, throat, or groin. When people surrounding you want to invade your country you develop a deadly art. Krav maga is not unlike the Marine Corps Martial Arts Program.

Silat is another violent hand-to-hand combat form.[23] Developed in the region of Southeast Asia, specifically Malaysia, it is identified by swift attack styles meant to close on the opponent quickly. Malaysia was a brutalized country invaded by pirates, the Portuguese, and the Japanese. Silat was developed to repel invaders. Like all hand-to-hand combat martial arts, fairness is dispensed with in favor of efficiency. In Southeast Asia, the martial arts also favor knife fighting.

Escrima is a Southeast Asian art that originated in the Philippines. It employs sticks and knives as the weapons of choice.[24] In 1521, Spanish explorer Ferdinand Magellan was hacked to death by Filipino natives. The knife fighting portion of the art is especially brutal and effective. The knives used in these fights were designed specifically for efficiency.

Jujutsu is one of the oldest close combat arts.[25] It was developed by Samurai in the Sengoku period to defeat armored enemies. Throws, joint locks, and striking in vital areas proved more effective than striking the armor of an opponent. This Japanese approach differed from neighboring China and Okinawa, which favored strictly striking techniques. Striking in jujutsu was as much a distracting technique to unbalance the opponent leading up to a joint lock or throw. Using an opponent's energy against him was also a key feature. As time progressed, judo, aikido, and other arts were derived from jujutsu methods. This is not to be confused with Brazilian jiu-jitsu, which is an offshoot of Japanese jujutsu. Brazilian methods emphasize grappling techniques on the ground.

In Japan, the Samurai played for keeps. Their techniques were designed to disable or kill an opponent. Jujutsu was not developed for sport.

Notice the common denominator of the most successful ancient leaders or effective martial arts styles. Each incorporated the basic principles of winning fights, including principles that may seem uncivilized or difficult. In addition to specific leaders and general martial arts approaches, there are also groups of warriors who were known for their fierce fighting.

FEROCIOUS GROUPS

The Samurai comprise the most obvious fierce group. They lived by the bushido code of the warrior and were bound by honor. Their feudal Ninja counterparts were fierce as well.[26] Ninja contrasted a bit with the Samurai in that their approach was to utilize anything that worked, including unorthodox methods. They were essentially spies and assassins, and some Samurai became Ninja warriors.

Lesser-known fierce warriors were the Maori of New Zealand.[27] They have been called the unforgiving fierce slayers of the South Seas. The Maori settled in the area around 1280 CE and believed *manna* or respect could only be gained from ancestors or combat. They developed fortified villages called *pa* and reportedly had a reputation for eating their enemies to capture their manna, which was spiritual power to them.[28] The Maori were never conquered and still exist today. Their native culture is slipping away through modernization. Some Maori serve in the New Zealand military.

The Zande tribe in Central Africa would sharpen their teeth to appear as cannibals to their enemies.[29] They were known for their brutality and took no prisoners during battles. The tribe still exists today along with another African tribe known as the Zulu. In the 1800s, under the fierce African warlord Shaka Zulu, they reportedly killed 2 million of their enemies, thus transforming the continent. They killed their enemies down to the last fighter. They were known as the Spartans of Africa.

The ancient Spartans built the finest military organization of the ancient world through brutality and harshness that developed fierce warriors.[30] Like the Samurai, the Spartans held to a strict code of honor. Military training began in adolescence and Spartans were lifelong soldiers. A lower class of skilled laborers and craftsmen took care of manufacturing and agriculture, leaving Spartan leaders to be preoccupied with the study of warfare.

Vikings were considered fierce warriors due to also having unorthodox fighting methods and extreme aggression.[31] They were particularly skillful in using the battle-axe. Knights in England were brave warriors as well.

The Apache were one of the fiercest tribes in North America.[32] There were seven major Apache tribes in the late 1800s. They had no rules for fighting other than to kill their enemies, which were typically surrounding Navajo and Comanche tribes. Scalping was a common practice to obtain as trophies from slain enemies.

By 1850, they began fighting Mexican and American soldiers. The leader during this time was the most famous warrior, Geronimo. After Mexican soldiers killed his family, Geronimo organized a force of 200 men and hunted down the Mexican soldiers and killed them. He was one of the last warriors to resist the government. He surrendered in 1886 with only about sixteen warriors left after being hunted by thousands of soldiers.

There are many more standout warriors throughout history. But the modern-day military Special Forces make up the current groups of fierce warriors. Each branch of the military has its own units that are specially trained and are the deadliest warriors to date. No warrior in history can match their current firepower and capabilities. With modern-day equipment and advances in methods backed by 2,500 years of proven principles of war, today's Special Forces operators are essentially unstoppable, limited only by the rules imposed upon them by nonwarrior political leaders. There is no doubt that current Special Forces operators are the fiercest warriors to date, as no group in history can match the violence they are able to deliver.

IN THE DOJO

Finishing second for the silver medal spot in the National Black Belt Leagues (NBL) World Championships held in Houston, Texas, many years ago was a martial arts tournament career highlight. The year before, the highlight was a Self-Defense Division First Place win in the Sport Karate Amateur International (SKIL) World Championships in Panama City, Florida.

The finish in the NBL Self-Defense Division in Texas came after a perfect season of 10 first-place wins on the East Coast. Martial arts always has an East Coast versus West Coast rivalry. Chuck Norris was a West Coast martial artist. His biggest rival was East Coast martial artist Joe Lewis. It was always an honor to represent your coast when two champions went head to head. But that's not the point.

The point is that competitors demonstrated hand-to-hand combat techniques in tournament play based on scoring. While other martial artists were doing some great kicks, punches, and a few assorted combat techniques, all our training was combat-ending moves that were brief, quick, and fight finishing. There seemed to be fewer being that aggressive in tournament style competitions in those days.

We tried to be fierce. All our moves were designed to disable, maim, and even kill. Marines watched us demonstrate at a tournament near Camp Lejeune, North Carolina, early in the season. They loved what we were doing and recognized the techniques as mirroring their own hand-to-hand combat. Shouts of "Hooah!" resonated throughout the arena whenever we performed for U.S. Marines.

These competitions took place years before movies like *The Bourne Identity* and *John Wick* would showcase these techniques in life-or-death struggles on the screen. At the time, having fierce moves designed only to disable was a novel approach. Elbows, knees, throat strikes, and groin kicks along with throws and arm locks were among our bag of techniques. It was nothing fancy—just hard-hitting, close-up combat. We'd get bloody just doing demonstrations. It was fierce.

In retrospect, it was the style of martial art being presented that consistently won those tournaments rather than simply our individual talent, as many on our team would consistently win tournament self-defense divisions. Judges loved the realism brought to that division and other winners had gradually been bringing that realism before us, as we weren't the first. You couldn't demonstrate those techniques anywhere else. The moves were not permitted in any other venue, and even in our venue we demonstrated them and held back before the ending joint breaks or killing moves for scoring. It was something new to many, much like the Bourne movies brought martial arts film into a new era of realism that was devoid of fake wires and shaky camera techniques. We tried to demonstrate technique as close to real as we could demonstrate it without killing someone or breaking things very much.

In one such demonstration the action was quick. My black gi was drenched in sweat as I demonstrated techniques for the audience on a team of ukes. *Uke* is a Japanese term commonly used in aikido, meaning a martial arts partner who acts as an opponent.

Our art, ketsugo do jujutsu, was simply an eclectic school of early traditional Japanese jujutsu practiced by the Samurai. There are many hand-to-hand combat forms derived from the original classical jujutsu. The crowd enjoyed the intensity of the action, quick throws, and rapid technique. At the end of the demonstration, I threw the final uke then flipped him onto his abdomen by straightening out his arm before jumping on his back to simulate breaking the arm. But before getting off the uke, I grabbed his hair and pulled his head back. With my other hand under his chin I let both hands slip quickly off the sides of his head in opposite directions without moving his head. I then yelled. Had I held on to his head the motion would have been deadly, but few noticed as the demonstration was over after I let out a scream ending the head technique.

The crowd cheered. Nearby black belts clapped but they had noticed the final technique and with understanding seemed to clap more nervously. The technique simulated snapping the opponent's neck. We had talked about whether to demonstrate such ferocity publicly. Many spectators of tournaments may not understand the full range of capabilities and the extreme violence that can be delivered. Master Miller authorized the demonstration, as it was what we did, so why not exhibit the full array? Earlier in the demonstration were eye gouges, throat strikes, and not just striking the groin but grabbing and simulating tearing out the groin. The demonstrations were meant to show the brutality of the art. These moves tended to get a lot of attention.

A tournament official smiled and leaned toward me after I helped my uke get up off the floor. "You know you guys are crazy, don't you?" she asked.

Our techniques had been called barbarous in the past. Our fighters had always been told that we all fought dirty. While most other martial arts schools were wearing white uniforms, our black belts wore all black. The stark difference in our approach to fighting seemed to extend beyond the color difference in our attire. Though many other schools taught similar techniques only a few demonstrated hand-to-hand brutality in public. The brutality of the techniques probably did seem crazy. But they were designed for combat. They were brutally effective. The methods were fierce and realistic. This wasn't martial arts for sport, and if you are a fighter it is the approach to take in order to win a fight.

In retrospect, that was the essence of the success of hand-to-hand combat techniques from war to tournament demonstrations. Effective fighting technique has an element of crazy aggression that seems barbarous and wild to the observer. To the outsider, only a maniac would have no rules in a fight. Techniques designed to end the fight quickly by any means seemed over the top and maybe ungentlemanly as well. But though it is brutal, it is effective.

When we talk about being fierce, the mental image is of an aggressive fighter punching and kicking, as seen on TV. The fight looks clean. But that's not how it is in real life and that isn't the full scale of fierce aggression. It will get you called crazy even in a martial arts tournament and is the kind of ferocious application of technique that wins.

Some martial artists demonstrated the full brutality of hand-to-hand combat technique before we did. But it's difficult to simulate in those venues. In a real fight, a fierce fighter will execute every bone-crunching, eye-gouging, groin-tearing, neck-breaking, and throat-striking technique at his disposal if that is what is necessary to survive. But shear brutality is what a fierce fight looks like.

FIERCE EXTREMES

While fierce means a lot of things, such as being aggressive and ruthless, maybe there is the appearance of uncontrolled madness in it as well. It's probably the impression we gave in demonstrations years ago. But there is a useful method at work when being fierce appears to be madness. It is the principle of focus that channels this otherwise maniacal madness and creates a sense of cool professionalism to end fights and instill fear within potential opponents. That is how to be ferocious and is essential to professionals in the fight business.

Movies like *The Bourne Identity* and *John Wick* have now moved these realistic demonstrations of fierce fighting to the screen. Fierce aggression wins fights.

While this fierce behavior must be tempered according to the situation, it is a principle that marks the greatest warriors, styles, and groups of fighters in history. Fierce fighters have this combination of behaviors or willingness to engage to whatever extreme is necessary to win.

The image of being fierce isn't necessarily pleasant. But it's necessary to win.

NOTES

1. Mike Adams, "Gandhi Advocated the Right to Bear Arms; Use 'Violence' to Defend Innocents Against Bullying, Oppression," *Natural News.com*, December 17, 2012, http://www.naturalnews.com/038372_Gandhi_nonviolence _right_to_bear_arms.html.

2. Dan Marcou, "Why Cops Should be Dangerous," *Policeone.com*, February 14, 2013, https://www.policeone.com/police-jobs-and-careers/articles/6116295 -Why-cops-should-be-dangerous/.

3. Thomas Michie, *Encyclopedia of the United States Supreme Court Reports* (Charlottesville, VA: The Michie Company Law Publishers), 542–543.

4. Steve Rowe, "The Martial Arts and Violence," *SteveRoweCom Blog*, November 19, 2015, https://steve-rowe.com/2015/11/19/the-martial-arts-and-violence/.

5. Jordan Harms, "Reagan's Inspiring Words on Defense: 'Peace Through Strength,'" *Daily Signal*, April 1, 2013, http://dailysignal.com/2013/04/01 /reagans-inspiring-words-on-defense-peace-through-strength/.

6. John Heubusch, "Peace Through Strength, Across Centuries: True Then, True Today," *National Interest*, August 29, 2016, http://nationalinterest.org/blog /the-buzz/peace-through-strength-across-the-centuries-true-then-true-17511.

7. Smithsonian, "Boeing B-29 Superfortress 'Enola Gay,'" *National Air and Space Museum*, n.d., https://airandspace.si.edu/collection-objects/boeing-b-29 -superfortress-enola-gay.

8. James Wright and Peter Rossi, *Armed Criminals in America: A Survey of Incarcerated Felons* (Boston: Social and Demographic Research Institute United States of America, 1985), 27–29, https://www.ncjrs.gov/App/Publications /abstract.aspx?ID=97099.

9. "Text of Churchill's Speech on War Prospects," *New York Times*, January 21, 1940, Page 30, Column 4, http://query.nytimes.com/gst/abstract.html?res=9E 03E5D7113EE23ABC4951DFB766838B659EDE&legacy=true.

10. Sun Tzu, *The Art of War and Other Classics of Eastern Thought* (New York: Barnes & Noble, 2013).

11. Steven Reddy, "Dying for Control: The Motivation of a Serial Killer," *Linked-In Blog*, March 10, 2015, https://www.linkedin.com/pulse/dying-control -motivation-serial-killer-steven-reddy.

12. Gavin Becker, *The Gift of Fear* (New York: Random House, 1997).

13. *John Wick*, written by Derek Kolstad, directed by Chad Stahelski and David Leitch (2014).

14. Ivan Bilibin, "Baba Yaga," *Old Russia.net*, n.d., http://www.oldrussia.net/baba .html.

15. Lucas Johnson, "Awesome Facts about Keanu Reeves' John Wick," *Movie Pilot Blog* (2015), https://moviepilot.com/posts/2669003.

16. Benjamin Griffin, "What Does John Wick's Tattoo Mean?" *Quora Blog*, September 20, 2016, https://www.quora.com/What-do-John-Wicks-tattoos-mean.

17. Rick Calvert, "Greek Thoughts," *Studylight.org*, n.d., http://classic.studylight .org/col/ds/.

18. History.com, "Genghis Khan," *A&E Network* (2009), http://www.history .com/topics/genghis-khan.

19. Steven Pinker, *The Better Angels of Our Nature: Why Violence Has Declined* (New York: Penguin, 2012).

20. "Ming Dynasty," *Encyclopædia Britannica* (2015), https://www.britannica .com/topic/Ming-dynasty-Chinese-history.

21. History.com, "Alexander the Great," *A&E Network*, n.d., http://www.his tory.com/topics/ancient-history/alexander-the-great.

22. Izhac Grinberg, "Israeli Martial Arts: A Brief Timeline," *Tactica Krav Maga Institute*, April 20, 2014, http://www.kravmagainstitute.com/instructor-develop ment/history-of-krav-maga/.

23. Brad Curran, "Martial Art of the Month: Silat," *Kung Fu Kingdom.com* (2015), http://kungfukingdom.com/martial-art-of-the-month-silat/.

24. Julius Melegrito, "Ten Things You Probably Didn't Know about the Filipino Martial Arts," *Black Belt Magazine*, January 24, 2017.

25. Robert Rousseau, "The History and Style of Japanese Jujutsu," *ThoughtCo* (2017), https://www.thoughtco.com/history-and-style-guide-jujutsu-2308254.

26. Kallie Szczepanski, "The Ninja of Japan," *ThoughtCo* (2017), https://www .thoughtco.com/history-of-the-ninja-195811.

27. Ministry for Culture and Heritage, "Polynesian Explorers," *New Zealand History*, March 7, 2014, https://nzhistory.govt.nz/culture/explorers/polynesian -explorers.

28. Yulia Dzhak, "Legendary Warriors—The Maori 'I Will Kill You and I Will Eat You,'" *War History Online* (2016), https://www.warhistoryonline.com/history /legendary-warriors_maori.html.

29. T. L. Jeffcoat, "Weapons & Warriors: The Living Nightmares of the Congo," *MrTalksTooMuch Blogspot*, April 25, 2012, http://mrtalkstoomuch.blogspot .com/2012/04/zande-warriors-living-nightmares-of.html.

30. History.com, "Sparta," *A&E Network* (2009), http://www.history.com/topics /ancient-history/sparta.

31. Emma Mason, "A Brief History of the Vikings," *History Extra*, May 25, 2016, http://www.historyextra.com/article/feature/brief-history-vikings-facts.

32. PBS.org, "Apache Warriors," *History Detectives*, n.d., http://www.pbs.org/opb /historydetectives/feature/apache-warriors/.

敬馬

リーダ・武蔵

SURPRISE

THE PROBLEM WITH most texts on warfare, such as Sun Tzu's, is that they tell you to use surprise, but they don't tell you how. There is a huge gap in knowledge of how some principles like surprise actually work.

Surprise is the first principle of offensive encounters. However, in defensive encounters it is the last, as it is usually relinquished to the aggressor.

But if the other principles are implemented with enough vigor, the element of surprise is attained even when in a defensive posture. This catches the attacker off guard. Many times an aggressor will not anticipate a calculated aggressive response. Doing what the aggressor doesn't expect helps a fighter attain the element of surprise. So there is always this struggle over who will achieve the element of surprise in a fight, as it is so powerful.

There are stories of potential victims feigning a seizure or pretending not to understand English and a host of other unexpected responses to an attack that surprised an aggressor. Any response other than an expected response will throw off an aggressor.

Surprise can be described as a strategic element meant to amaze, overwhelm, ambush, or bewilder. The principle is so important that a smaller force can overcome a much larger force if it is used effectively.

The first two principles of preparation and awareness help counter the element of surprise. These first two principles are the first line of defense against surprise in any form.

The first application that comes to mind regarding surprise is in offensive operations, as in setting up an ambush or striking at an unexpected time or place. Offensive applications of this element are easier to envision. When surprise penetrates preparation and awareness it is difficult to counter.

DEFENSIVE SURPRISE

One observer of violence once suggested that when faced with the scenario of a home invasion where the intruders held a weapon to a child demanding the rest of the family sit down to be tied up, that an option was for one of the other members to immediately escape.[1] While initially this advice sounds horrific as the child is being left to the mercy of the intruders, there is an interesting rationale for this reaction's success.

The escape of another family member means the clock is suddenly ticking for the intruders. Help will soon be on the way. The author of this solution rationalizes that if the intruders harm the child then they were going to harm everyone anyway. A family member suddenly running away rather than complying with the threat of harm to the child introduces the element of surprise. It changes the dynamic. It alters the control the intruders initially achieved.

The same thought is true for running away from someone with a gun. If the aggressor shoots the victim in the back as he runs, he was probably going to shoot the victim anyway. It is difficult to ascertain if this is true in all instances. But these are interesting examples of surprising an aggressor.

Many years ago the standard police tactic for certain situations was to form a perimeter, keep the suspects pinned inside the perimeter, and negotiate with them as a specially trained SWAT team was put in place.[2] The shootings at Columbine High School changed everything and the rise of terrorist activity put an exclamation point to the change. Now training involves the first officers on the scene confronting active shooter suspects immediately and aggressively. Active threats like active shooters must be differentiated from potential threats like hostage takers.

An effective enemy ambush tactic is to place an obstacle on a road that allows the ambushing forces to hide and cause their victims to stop in front of them. Land mines are planted in the ditches on either side of the road where the ambushed soldiers might attempt to gain cover once they stop for the obstacle and begin to be engaged by the enemy.[3] Snipers can then be placed on either side to pick off any soldiers the mines do not eliminate. This surrounds the intended victims on three sides.

If you ask the average person what would you do if enemy soldiers popped up behind an obstacle across a road and began firing at your squad of men, the natural answer would be to immediately dive for cover in the ditches to each side. But a seasoned soldier would realize a well-planned ambush would anticipate this move and place explosives in the ditches or have snipers in place.

A seasoned soldier's answer would be different. If faced with such a scenario, the better choice may be for the squad to immediately attack the enemy head on and quickly. You would have more men to mount a counterattack that focuses on one spot head-on and achieves the element of surprise.

The 1776 Battle of Trenton is one of the most famous surprise attacks in U.S. history. General George Washington crossed the icy Delaware River on Christmas night, leading 2,400 Continental Army troops on an unexpected raid against British-supported German Hessian mercenaries garrisoned at Trenton, New Jersey.[4] The surprise raid had a lasting effect.

DEFINING SURPRISE

The distinction between the tactical and strategic applications of surprise is vague. Sometimes this differentiation is the scale of surprise. And although the aggressor gets the first shot at surprise, the way it's achieved is the same on both sides. So we'll tackle it all at once.

To produce surprise requires the opponent to form a preconception of intentions and capabilities of his victim, target, or even nation (or you as the other fighter in a sports match). This can be set up by deception, whereby one fighter deliberately misleads his opponent in some manner. This counters the aggressor's advantage of having surprise on his side, since the aggressor gets to choose the timing for the most part.

Timing is the element the aggressor wields. The other fighter's actual response must be secret and not telegraphed in advance. This is the deceptive element. But when the counter response is launched, it must be swift. The idea is that one side fools the other side. Deception works on both sides by any manner.

The idea of one side being surprised by the capabilities or actions of the other can be translated on any scale including war. Surprise on either side of the equation means that something unexpected happened. One side has deceived the other.

Surprise doesn't win a fight all by itself, but it does provide a huge advantage to the fighter who uses it. The window of opportunity of that advantage is slim, as the opponent will soon recover. Based on this, the four factors that produce strategic surprise are:[5,6]

1. Secrecy
2. Deception
3. Preconception
4. Timing

Creating surprise in a defensive posture is difficult, as the four elements are best utilized for offensive surprise. Unexpected action when attacked achieves this defensive adaptation of surprise.

Keeping capabilities or actions secret, deceiving the opponent, taking advantage of preconceived notions and bias, or choosing the timing of attacks or unexpected responses are key ways to execute this principle.

Surprise is a force multiplier. If it can be achieved in the defensive posture its effects are even more devastating, as the opponent had preconceived notions and must readapt to the situation. Do not think all is lost if surprise penetrates your preparation and awareness. But it does increase the odds of winning, even if ever so briefly.

APPLICATIONS

A weapon is an example of a force multiplier. Imagine an attacker trying to rob a victim with a knife. The intended victim then pulls out a gun. The gun is a force multiplier as well. Only it is a bigger force multiplier. This increased force introduced into the situation achieves surprise even in the defensive posture. But naturally, surprise is even more effective in the offensive posture.

Military strategists have long adhered to the 3 to 1 doctrine of a successful attack.[7] Commanders prefer a 3 to 1 superiority of force during an offensive action. Guerrilla warfare, in which the enemy strikes then hides within a peaceful populace, has injected surprise to upset this doctrine many times throughout history. Patriots during the American Revolution used the tactic, as did the Vietcong and most recently Middle Eastern terrorists.

In the defensive posture a bigger gun (a force multiplier that evens the odds) or a bigger surprise (guerrilla warfare) levels the playing field. In the offensive posture, surprise alone can be successful. It's just easier to pull off in the offensive posture.

Much has been learned about the effectiveness of surprise by studying past wars. A surprise location of attack typically leads the list as the most successful type of surprise, followed by timing, strength assessments, intention, and style of attack.[8] You can see how there are parallels on the scale of personal attacks as well. Uncertainty is an effective tool in winning.

Offensive surprise is a much easier tactic and leads the way surprise is strategically implemented in war regarding location and timing. Defensive surprise is a bit trickier and must counter with force multipliers, intention, or style of response to create the same effective surprise as offensive actions.

Offensive attacks have the advantage of picking the location and time of attack. But the lesser-used surprise methods of strength (force), failure of the aggressor to assess the victim's capabilities, or style of response by the victim or target have strategic value in a defensive posture. All these methods of introducing uncertainty apply universally.

The importance of surprise to an individual fighter is removing your opponent's advantage of uncertainty by preparation and awareness. Surprise can be incorporated into your own fight game by doing the unexpected or injecting other elements for which the opponent is unprepared. The bottom line is that anything utilized for which the opponent is unprepared achieves surprise.

In this sense, the principle of surprise is achieved if the attack or counterattack secures an advantage against an opponent who has inadequate defenses or is unprepared. This allows some wiggle room between offensive and defensive surprise, which is always the problem. Surprise only works if the opponent has not prepared and is not aware. It works both ways. The amount of preparation and awareness determines the amount of effect surprise will achieve in either direction. That's the wiggle room either side has in countering or achieving surprise. Surprise is successful not simply because it occurs, but because it achieves advantage by an action resulting from its use. This could be a surprise attack or a surprise response to an attack. The amount of preparation of either fighter determines the differences in the amount of success this surprise will achieve if accompanied by an effective action. That is the variability of surprise.

Surprise can also be achieved not by the absence of an opponent's awareness, but in spite of it. This is where the element of deception is injected best. Any gap in knowledge the opponent has regarding the fighter can be exploited for surprise. It may be an underestimation of capabilities, timing, or some other factor. Gaps in warning time or gaps in knowledge are where the injection of surprise is successful.

While war doctrines approach surprise in fighting as a cross between speed and secrecy, it should be viewed in terms of information versus no information. If you have a lot of information through awareness then it is almost impossible for you to be surprised. But if you are unaware with little information you will always be surprised. Injecting false information into the other fighter's awareness structure is an effective technique.

Over the millennia there have been many writings utilizing surprise as a fighting doctrine. Specifically, Sun Tzu discussed the importance of surprise 2,000 years ago. The Roman diplomat Frontinus (c. 75 CE) indicated in his prolific writings that surprise is achieved by attacking weakness or to attack where unexpected, with the unexpected, and when unexpected.[9]

The Romans expanded on this thought around 390 CE when Publius Flavius Vegetius Renatus wrote that it is better to overcome an enemy by famine, surprise, or terror than with general actions.[10] Views on surprise haven't changed but its application has varied somewhat.

EXPLOITATION

More recent military scholars added more specific views on secrecy and deception. Some were skeptical that surprise was even possible in a more advanced technological age. Wilhelm von Leeb and Carl von Clausewitz agreed that speed was an excellent tactic to execute surprise in battle.[11] But they added exploitation as an element. In other words, there must be strong action coupled with surprise or else it is no different than jumping out from behind a bush and yelling, "Boo!"

To fully exploit the value of surprise, there must be substance in terms of a goal. Otherwise, an opponent will quickly realize he has been caught off guard and will correct the problem. A fighter must not only surprise but must fully exploit the brief advantage it provides. Surprise must be quickly followed by a substantial plan of action to fully benefit from the principle with a goal in mind.

Again, the successful elements of surprise are achieved if the action is unexpected. This includes location, timing, style, method, and size of attack, or any approach that violates the opponent's assumptions or expectations. This must be coupled with no advance warning and executed quickly enough to prevent a countersurprise. The opposition must not see the real thing coming. Exploitation must occur quickly as well. Surprise is a powerful principle but there is a small window of opportunity available to take full advantage of its strength. This is why you must know what you wish to achieve by its use—then, do it quickly.

ACTIONS FOLLOW DECISIONS

Awareness of surprise not only means being alert, as deception can exploit watchfulness. Therefore, you must understand a rule. The rule is that actions are the result of decisions, not the other way around.

Whether it is something as small as someone crossing the street toward you or as large as a buildup of military units on a border, don't assume you cannot discern intentions. Begin to account for any connections that may explain the action. Don't assume the action is conducted without any plan in mind. Don't assume the action is waiting on a decision, because if you see an action the plan has already been decided. The plan may be peaceful or the plan may be violent.

When something unusual occurs, ask yourself: What does this action suggest about the opponent's plans? People seldom do things without a purpose, especially in a fight. It is too risky to do otherwise.

If an army is forming at a border, intelligence analysts don't assume they are just forming there waiting on a decision. They assume a decision has been made and the action is a result of a decision.

Pay attention to what people do, not what they say. What they say may be setting up surprise through deception. Pay attention to actions. Notice those who do not applaud when you win. Seek out those who motivate, inspire, and stick with you when you lose. This differentiates those who will surprise you from those who will not.

Surprise is a powerful principle. Intervening before someone surprises you can occur if you already know the opponent. Countering with your own surprise thwarts an unknown opponent. Preparation and awareness are the enemies of surprise but awareness can be fooled. Pay close attention to the actions of those around you, not their words, and do not assume actions are meaningless waiting on a decision, because nothing occurs without first a thought or a plan. Actions always follow decisions, not the other way around.

These are ways to combat surprise and execute surprise, because surprise is brief but powerful. But remember, surprise must be coupled with an action.

NOTES

1. Sam Harris, "The Truth about Violence," *Sam Harris Blog*, n.d., http://www .samharris.org/blog/item/the-truth-about-violence.
2. Police Executive Research Forum, "The Police Response to Active Shooter Incidents," *PoliceForum.org*, March 2014, http://www.policeforum.org/assets /docs/Critical_Issues_Series/the%20police%20response%20to%20active%20 shooter%20incidents%202014.pdf.
3. Hans Halberstadt, *U.S. Navy Seals* (St. Paul, MN: Zenith Press, 2006), 9.
4. History.com, "Battles of Trenton and Princeton" (2009), http://www.history .com/topics/american-revolution/battles-of-trenton-and-princeton.
5. Maj. Jack H. Spencer, "Deception Integration in the U.S. Army," master's thesis, California State Polytechnic University, 1974, http://www.dtic.mil/dtic/tr /fulltext/u2/a230184.pdf.

6. Cynthia Grabo, "Anticipating Surprise: Analysis for Strategic Warning," *Center for Strategic Intelligence Research: Joint Military Intelligence College* (2002), http://www.ni-u.edu/ni_press/pdf/Anticipating_Surprise_Analysis.pdf.
7. Moshe Kress and I. Talmor, "A New Look at the 3:1 Rule of Combat Through Markov Stochastic Lanchester Models," *Journal of Operational Research Society* 50 (1999): 733–744.
8. Meir Finkel, *On Flexibility: Recovery from Technological and Doctrinal Surprise on the Battlefield* (Palo Alto, CA: Stanford University Press), 23–35.
9. Sextus Frontinus, "Strategems," Loeb Classics Library (1925), https://www.loebclassics.com/view/frontinus-stratagems/1925/pb_LCL174.205.xml.
10. Flavius Renatus, *The Military Institutions of the Romans* (Morrisville, NC: Lulu Press, 2017), 66; Robert Nelson, *Inspirational Lessons from Inspirational People* (Morrisville, NC: Lulu Press, 2012).
11. Carl von Clausewitz, *On War* (1832), http://slantchev.ucsd.edu/courses/ps143a/readings/Clausewitz%20-%20On%20War,%20Books%201%20and%208.pdf.

時
判
日
断
寺
機

リーダー武蔵

TIMING

STRIKING AT THE RIGHT TIME is the essence of timing. There is a window of opportunity in a fight. A fighter must learn to seize opportunity when the moment presents itself. Timing is making the judgment that a certain action should be taken and then controlling when it is executed along with the tempo or pace at which it is executed.

It is fitting that timing follows surprise. Traditional U.S. Army counter-insurgency literature has long recognized the elements of an offensive action:

1. Surprise
2. Audacity
3. Timing
4. Concentration

We've discussed achieving surprise by striking at a time, place, or manner for which the opponent is unprepared. This lack of preparation may be the result of effective deception tactics that have convinced your opponent to make the wrong choice. In the U.S. Civil War, Union Army General William Sherman referred to this concept as putting your enemy on the horns of a dilemma and impaling him on the horn of your choosing.[1] Sherman is well known for his effective use of these offensive action elements.

Audacity is a simple plan, boldly executed, and timing the action so that the opponent cannot defend effectively.[2] Timing is a key component of pulling off a successful fight and delivering the other elements. Concentration is amassing forces for military operations or focusing power in individual confrontations.

Fight sequences are all about timing decisions. U.S. Air Force Colonel John Boyd was a Korean War veteran and a military strategist. He noted common denominators that occurred during war that spelled success or failure. His theories about these similarities influenced not only the Pentagon where he served as a consultant but sports and business as well.

As described earlier, Colonel Boyd became known for the OODA (Observation–Orientation–Decision–Action) Loop, which described his observations of many battles and their common factors.[3] Its application is even more evident in the principle of timing.

As we've seen, his view was that the winner of a fight would be determined by who could create situations where one could make better decisions more quickly than the other. Timing was key to this loop. All fighters go through this decision-making loop naturally. The theory is that whoever goes through the loop in the shortest time will prevail. As noted by Harry Hillaker, the chief designer of the F-16 fighter jet, the quickest thinker will always have an advantage as the opponent will still be responding to situations that have already changed. Hillaker was making the point that a smart fighter is making decisions faster than his opponent. This creates a situation where the successful fighter is several steps ahead of an opponent, who is responding to conditions that have already changed.

Much of Boyd's theory came from his students' notes. Boyd apparently didn't write much down. But many have referred to his idea as getting inside the head of an adversary by understanding what your adversary is doing, determining his intent, and interrupting his decisions before they become actions. Recall in our discussion on surprise that actions follow decisions. Smart timing interrupts the opponent during the decision-making process.

Let's say you are standing in front of a store. You see a couple of thugs approaching who seem to be looking at you. You have entered the first phase of the loop—**Observation.**

Entering the second phase (**Orientation**), you look around. The building is behind you. A semi-busy street is in front of you. Few people are on the street. The nearest door to the building seems open at first glance. Next to you is a newsstand. You step back a bit so that the building is behind you and the newsstand is to your side between you and the thugs. You are already setting up a plan whether anything happens or not.

The thugs stop in front of you. The newsstand is between you and one of them, who begins to scan the area nervously. The other thug says he needs your wallet. You then enter phase three of the loop (**Decision**) by deciding to maybe give them your wallet if they back off but you will attack if they exhibit any violent signals. You've already planned your attack if that becomes necessary.

The thug asking for the wallet then says he will just cut you and take the wallet, as you don't seem to be moving fast enough for him. He begins to reach into his pocket. Entering the last phase of the loop (**Action**), you deliver a blow to his throat then turn the newsstand over in front of the second thug. You then spin toward the door of the store, entering it quickly, moving into the store to escape out another door or find help inside.

You just went through an OODA loop. Understand that according to Boyd's theory, so did the thugs. They observed you as their target. They looked around orienting themselves to the prospect of robbing you. They made their decision and approached. Remember that action follows decision, not the other way around. But just as one of them began to act on the decision to commit a crime, you unexpectedly delivered a blow to the throat of one and temporarily blocked the path of the second before disappearing.

The thugs then had to go through another OODA loop because you interrupted their first loop. They started their plan over. While one is choking, the other is observing his friend choke while stepping over the newsstand. They both had to orient themselves to the situation they were now in while noting you had fled. They then have to make a decision to either pursue or flee. Interrupting their feedback loop gives you an advantage. Being able to go through a feedback loop to make decisions quicker than the opponent helps win fights, and timing is a key component of completing that loop.

Most fighters focus on action. But knowing when to bring an action into play is critical to winning the fight. The OODA loop is a decision-making process. Boyd believed the most effective organizations have a highly decentralized command structure with objective-driven goals rather than goals that are method driven to allow rapid OODA loop processing to respond to challenges. They are then able to time decisions accordingly and quickly.

Boyd based his theory on other important principles, such as Godel's incompleteness theory in which any model of reality is not complete as models must be continually adapting or changing in light of new observations. Boyd also noted Heisenberg's uncertainty principle, which describes the limit of our ability to precisely observe reality. Boyd's underlying belief was that survival depended on adapting to change and not on adapting to existing circumstances.[4]

Reducing the time spent on OODA loops and minimizing the number of loops to reach a goal is therefore key to winning a fight. Making your opponent burn up time dealing with loops interrupts their timing and gives you an edge to winning.

OPTIONS

In 2000, psychologists Sheena Iyengar and Mark Lepper published an interesting study that concluded that more options aren't always better.[5] They set up a display with 24 varieties of jelly. On another day they displayed only 6 varieties.

The large display attracted a lot of interest. But fewer people purchased from the larger display even though there were more options.

This study has been successfully reproduced many times in other fields. People simply don't make better decisions just because they have more options. They actually tend to make better decisions when given a smaller range of choices. It is called "choice paralysis." Imagine the martial artist who knows many techniques but has to go through a mental loop of which technique to employ versus a martial artist who is skilled in a few vital techniques.

These studies by psychologists and observations by Lee have to do with the Hick-Hyman Law. William Edmund Hick and Ray Hyman were

British and American psychologists who first noted these issues about choice in 1951.[6,7] They observed the time it took an individual to make a decision based on available choices. Increasing the choices increased the time to make a decision. More recent studies, such as those by Iyengar and Lepper, not only confirm this as a law of reaction time but also solidify the concept that information overloads can be paralyzing.

You may know a thousand punches. But if you have to think about which punch to use, then the guy who only knows one good punch will land his first and win. Choices and reaction time are all about timing. Simplicity can be your friend when it comes to timing.

SYNCHRONIZATION

We've noted that black belts strike hard not so much due to brute muscle strength as much as timing muscle movements in synchronous fashion for maximum striking potential. This is another aspect of timing. It is not so much what you do as how you are doing it and when you do it.

Sometimes it's just doing anything at all. A soccer ball kicked for a penalty shot takes about 0.3 seconds to reach the goal. One-third of the time a kicker kicks to the left, one-third to the right and one-third in the middle. This fraction of a second is really too quick for the goal keeper to watch the arc of the ball and make an accurate timing decision. So the player may dive to the right or left even if they are diving in the wrong direction. But if one-third of the time the ball is kicked in the middle, why doesn't the goal keeper just stand still if there is no statistical advantage to trying to time a leap in what may be the wrong direction? The player may move because inaction seems to be less acceptable than action. The player's timing is sometimes about appearance over effectiveness when you do the math over the timing decision. Society often rewards action over inaction—even if the action may be wrong. Fighters want to synchronize their timing for effective impact that is efficient and effective.

Even the fastest fighters are not always the winners. Though speed is essential, it is the fighter who is more efficient by hitting a weakness at an opportune moment. Speed wins fights but timing the speed wins more.

It simply builds upon other principles in order to apply them at the right time.

IN THE DOJO

Martial artists begin to exhibit a level of maturity when they begin to feel the tempo of a fight. A new student will jump in and out to land a punch or block a blow in awkward fashion when sparring for the first time.

But with time the student will begin to wait rather than rush the opponent. The student has learned to observe the opponent's movements, eyes, breathing, and footwork by taking it all in and striking during a moment the opponent is open or the opponent's guard is down, or sometimes counter punching as the opponent is recovering from an attack. Sometimes watching two black belts spar can be more boring to the casual observer. They may circle, dodge, and feign but there may be less action than when students spar. They are engaged in a chess match. The black belts are only striking when they feel the timing is right. They are constantly controlling the space between them until they determine the opportunity for a successful strike. There's more going on between them than it seems.

TIMING WORKS

Consider martial artists who continue to practice their art late in life. Many no longer have the strength or the speed. But their timing is impeccable, which makes up for the other factors. Timing allows actions to be more efficient by employing them at the right moment.

In 1809, Napoleon said that timing in war is the great element between weight and force. What he meant was that the most efficient use of time and resources was more important than conquering terrain in war.[8]

Time is the least forgiving element in a fight. The lack of some principles can be balanced by strength in others. But if timing is lacking, there are few other balancing options. It is not a neutral dimension. Weaknesses can be improved upon but if a fighter exhibits bad timing, time is something that is lost forever and can never be recovered. When you lose that moment of opportunity, that particular moment is gone.

Fighting involves hundreds of timing moments. Strength, speed, and other principles alone are important to delivering a fight. But knowing when to time the fight or when to strike is crucial to winning. Only experience and training can develop a sense of timing.

TIMING AS A PRINCIPLE

Quite frankly, when researching this book I viewed timing as a tactic, element, or variable needed to employ other principles. You will notice dozens of these smaller elements throughout the text. But upon having warriors review the principles it became clear that timing was a crucial principle itself in need of a bit more attention. It rose to the level of a broader principle.

When I asked a former marine what he thought of the principles and if there was anything in the text that needed a higher level of attention needed to win fights—he answered in one word: "Timing."

The discussion of timing in this chapter is from a broad perspective; timing as a strategic element that complements other principles. Then tempo is an even more intricate element in controlling the pace of the timing. Loren Christensen and Wim Demeere take a closer look at timing in their book, *Timing in the Fighting Arts*,[9] which is an examination of how fights are all about timing moments.

NOTES

1. William Sherman, *Memoirs of Gen. William T. Sherman* (New York: D. Appleton, 1891).
2. U.S. Department of the Army, *U.S. Army Counterinsurgency Warrior Handbook* (Lanham, MD: Rowman & Littlefield, 2015).
3. James Fallows, "John Boyd in the News: All You Need to Know about the OODA Loop," *The Atlantic*, August 29, 2015, https://www.theatlantic.com/notes/2015/08/john-boyd-in-the-news-all-you-need-to-know-about-ooda-loop/402847/.
4. "OODA Loop," Wikipedia, last modified June 25, 2017, https://en.wikipedia.org/wiki/OODA_loop.
5. Sheena Iyengar and Mark Lepper, "When Choice Is Demotivating: Can One Desire Too Much of a Good Thing?" *Journal of Personality and Social Psychology* 79 (2000): 995–1006.
6. T. Wu et al., "Hick-Hyman Law Is Mediated by the Cognitive Control Network in the Brain," *Cerebral Cortex* (May 22, 2017): 1–16.

7. Jed Brubaker, "Hick's Law," *Jed Brubaker Blog*, n.d., http://www.jedbrubaker .com/wp-content/uploads/2013/03/Day7-HicksLaw.pdf.
8. U.S. Army Center of Military History, *Historical Perspectives of the Operational Art*, edited by Michael Krause and Cody Phillips (Washington DC: Government Printing Office, 2006).
9. Loren Christensen and Wim Demeere, *Timing in the Fighting Arts* (Wolfeboro, NH: YMAA Publication Center, 2004).

堅忍

リーダー 武蔵

FORTITUDE

ULTIMATELY THERE MUST be the willingness to win. This must be coupled with a never-quit attitude. So while fortitude is having the mental and emotional strength to face adversity, it begins with willingness to win and ends with never giving up. It would seem obvious that a fighter would want to win. But if a fighter doesn't first have the will to win, he is doomed before he begins. A "never-give-up" attitude then finishes the winning task. Why wouldn't a fighter want to win?

This has been presented in many different ways in the literature. But the basic concept is that there are three levels to the thinking structure of the brain.

The first is basic survival; impulses such as hunger and fight or flight. Scientifically, this has been referred to as the triune brain or the reptilian complex[1] derived from the concept that these basic structures of thinking dominate in animals such as reptiles and birds.

The second level is a bit more complex and relates to the emotions. Mammals seem to have feelings more so than reptiles. Structures in the limbic system control mood, memory, and hormones.

The highest level is in the outer cortex and involves thinking that allows for complex social interactions and problem solving. How one reacts or handles situations is sometimes a construct of which level of thinking is being used.

The lowest reptilian areas of our brains are pretty good at basic survival, but are not able to solve problems at a high level. The second level is pretty good at social situations. But because this level relies heavily on emotion, it doesn't provide for good problem-solving skills requiring more complex thought. This results in conflict between how our emotional level and our highest levels of the brain each want to handle a problem.

For example, the second level, sometimes called the monkey brain, will tell us we can't win a fight. We aren't good enough. Now maybe it's right, but maybe it's lying to us because this level of thinking hates change. It's emotional.

Let's say you compose music but are afraid to play for anyone or audition for a show. The worst that can happen is that you would be rejected, and if your higher-level thinking were in play you'd realize not only is that not the end of the world, but that you might actually succeed. After all, you miss 100 percent of the shots you don't take. This type of thinking is called an irrational belief.

But your lower level of thinking is strictly emotional rather than logical. It not only fears failure but will fear success as well. If you were to succeed you might become famous and everything would change. The emotional level doesn't care if the change is good or bad. It just hates change.

In both instances, the monkey brain will act on emotion, telling you it can't be done. A fighter's own brain may be his worst enemy if it keeps telling him he can't win, he isn't good enough, or the fight is already lost.

This can be countered by engaging the higher levels of thinking that you possess. Think logically and practically. Think through a fight or conflict before it begins. Understand the possible solutions and outcomes of each solution.

Also, you must continually immerse yourself with positive input. Positive affirmations and inspirational messages help overcome or short circuit negative emotional responses. What you put in your brain will manifest itself in action. Fortitude is a positive attitude of never giving up the pursuit of the goal.

NEVER GIVE UP

There is a popular cartoon of a stork standing in a pond. In the stork's mouth are the legs of a frog the stork has just tried to eat. Although the rest of the frog's head and body are inside the stork's mouth, the frog has reached its arms outside the stork's beak with both hands wrapped firmly around the stork's throat. The stork's eyes are wide and its expression says that it doesn't know what to do. The caption reads, "never give up."

A fighter's toughest challenge is himself. We are our own biggest obstacles. Fighters must identify what these obstacles are and understand how they affect performance and perception of reality. This requires a higher level of thinking that rises above simple emotion.

Lack of commitment, lack of self-belief, faith, desire, or a hundred other obstacles can prevent success. Lacking the will power to persevere when these obstacles become tough is a constant challenge. Many of these challenges are internal and the result of what we tell ourselves. There is a constant dialogue in our brains that many refer to as self-talk. We can talk ourselves into and out of success. Internal obstacles are self-created and are the result of fear or emotions and are justified by excuses.

There are also external obstacles that are not self-created. This is why a fighter must have a strong belief system and build confidence each day to overcome both internal and external forces. You must tell yourself every day you are a winner. You must believe it yourself before anyone else is going to believe it.

If a fighter is focusing on obstacles, challenges, problems, or circumstances beyond the fighter's control then the focus isn't on what the fighter wants but on what the fighter doesn't want. This sabotages success by not focusing on the goal.

Every obstacle should act as a learning experience to drive the fighter closer to achieving the goal. Fighters should always remain optimistic and positive through each challenge. This should be reflected in the fighter's actions and words, as there are many Eastern and even Western religious schools of thought that mention speaking things into existence. Even language should be positively focused on the goal at hand. What you hear constantly and what you say constantly becomes reality. You become what you read and what you say.

An unstoppable attitude is vital to a fighter's success. Both thought and action should be optimistic, moving closer to the goal with each step. This creates momentum through sheer determination. Some call it having heart. It is a winning attitude.

A "never-give-up" attitude doesn't tackle a mountain all at one time because the obstacle is so enormous. There must be the determination to take one more step, then another and another, until finally the mountain is scaled, one step at a time.

Successful warriors commit themselves to a tangible goal. They then determine a plan to achieve that goal. Obstacles are simply viewed as stepping stones along the way and they never lose sight of the finish line. At the moment it seems a problem may swallow them, they grab it by the throat. They never give up.

GRIT

Another way of describing a "never-give-up" attitude is to use the concept called grit. While fortitude is the needed courage, bravery, backbone, and indomitable spirit necessary to face adversity, grit is the specific personal variable that gets it done.

A fighter with grit is passionate and driven by a powerful motivation to win. This motivation may be internally generated or external. But it creates a drive that is resilient.

Perseverance is one of the most powerful determinants of success. Resilience is a common personality trait among successful people who persevere over long periods of time to achieve a goal.

To achieve grit, a fighter must learn to manage fear of failure. Successful people actually embrace failure as part of the road to success. Michael Jordan is one of the most successful basketball players in history. He has said that he has missed over 9,000 shots in his career. He's lost hundreds of games and missed the winning shot on many of them. He has said that these failures are why he succeeds.[2]

Put simply, players miss 100 percent of the shots they never take. Everyone fails. The key is to take the shots, then keep trying until you reach the goal. That's grit. There is a story that illustrates this point nicely on how never quitting begins with deciding to start.

One day a man was visiting his elderly next-door neighbor. As they sat on the elderly man's front porch, the man noticed his neighbor's dog seemed to be resting comfortably between them, but would periodically moan softly. So he asked his neighbor why his dog was moaning. The elderly gentleman calmly responded that it was because his dog was lying on a nail in the porch. The man asked his neighbor why his dog didn't just get off the nail. "Because it doesn't hurt bad enough," was the elderly man's reply.

This is the problem of fortitude. Before having a spirit that never quits, there first must be the desire to get started. Something has to hurt bad enough or drive you hard enough to get off the nail, to take the shot and create the conditions you need to succeed. Do not get comfortable and fear that moving forward will be more uncomfortable. Fortitude is about internal drive. And internal drive is a predictor of success.

In 2006, the U.S. Navy Seals conducted a study titled, "Predictors of Success in Basic Underwater Demolition/SEAL (BUD/S) Training."[3] Researchers determined that among the factors that determined success in terms of human endurance in extreme environments was mental toughness. It explained why attempts at measuring a warrior's external factors were less accurate at predicting success in the most grueling training the military has to offer.

The guy who was 5 foot 5 and weighed 150 pounds soaking wet might make it through training while someone else, who was 6 foot 2 with a muscular physique and weighed 200 pounds, might not. It was what the fighter has inside that ultimately matters most. The size of the fighter doesn't equate to success. It is the size of the fighter's fortitude.

Best-selling author and psychologist Angela Duckworth conducted a study of West Point cadets in 2004. Her book, *Grit: The Power of Passion and Perseverance,* was a result of that work. She elaborates on the qualities that determine success. She called this measure grit. Her work determined that grit trumps IQ and talent, noting that although no one has figured out how to truly make someone smarter, the qualities of grit may be teachable. This is important to fighters because grit is what separates good from great.

FORTITUDE IN ACTION

This principle is embedded into the culture of current military warrior organizations. The last line of the U.S. Rangers' creed is, "Readily will I display the intestinal fortitude required to fight on to the Ranger objective and complete the mission though I be the lone survivor."[4]

A part of the U.S. Navy Seal code is, "Ready to lead, ready to follow, never quit."[5] The U.S. Army soldier's creed also includes a line about a soldier who will never quit. The airman's creed has a similar focus, stating an airman will never falter and will not fail. Every branch of military service honors this code. Fortitude is a warrior tradition. It is a winning principle. We also see it within successful people and successful organizations.

On December 22, 1944, the German army surrounded members of the U.S. 101st Airborne Division, who were defending the town of Bastogne, Belgium. This was the World War II Battle of the Bulge. Under a flag of truce, the German commander sent a letter to U.S. General Anthony McAuliffe informing him that a superior German force surrounded him and that if he did not surrender the Germans would attack. He was given two hours to respond.

General McAuliffe wasn't known to be a man to swear and it didn't take him two hours to make up his mind. Immediately, he had an aide type a reply that he sent back to the Germans. The note read:

December 22, 1944
To the German Commander,
N U T S!
The American Commander

General McAuliffe's nephew confirmed the story. The German commander at first did not understand the reply, asking if this was an affirmative or negative response. Private First Class Ernest Premetz was a German-speaking medic assigned to the U.S. platoon hosting the German officers who had delivered the note. Although the German officers spoke English, Premetz wanted to make sure they understood the U.S. commanders' response. In German, he told them the note meant for them to go to hell and if the Germans attacked they'd kill every one of them.[6]

The Germans did attack. But the American forces held the town until reinforcements arrived from the U.S. 4th Armored Division on December 26. The American victory at Bastogne helped ensure the final defeat of the German army.

There are countless stories of warriors never giving up. There are countless personal stories of soldiers wounded in battle and struggling to recover from their wounds through perseverance. Fortitude is ingrained in the warrior spirit.

In the martial arts, a black belt is not necessarily defined as someone who cannot be beaten in any given fight. Every fighter can be beaten on any given day. But a black belt is typically a fighter who will not give up easily. He may get knocked down, but he will keep getting back up if he can. And he will keep fighting. A black belt should personify the warrior spirit of never giving up.

VIRTUE

The four cardinal virtues in classical antiquity including theological traditions were prudence, justice, temperance, and courage.[7] In his work *The Republic*, Plato associated each virtue with a class of citizens.[8] Temperance was common to all classes according to his view. Prudence was a virtue assigned mostly to rulers, and justice was outside the class divisions of man. Courage was also described as fortitude and assigned to the warrior class.

In the view of most philosophers of antiquity, justice and prudence were virtues that helped people to determine what needed to be done. Fortitude was the virtue that provided the strength to do it.

There is a quote attributed to John Wayne: "Courage is being scared to death but saddling up anyway."[9] That is the essence of fortitude, which isn't the absence of fear but the persistent response to it.

MENTAL MUSCLE

Admiral William McRaven was a Navy Seal for 37 years. He is author of *Make Your Bed: Little Things That Can Change Your Life . . . and Maybe the World*.[10] He relates that it takes tremendous fortitude to survive Seal training. He says that the secret to success is refusing to quit.

If it were that easy everyone could do it. But McRaven says the key is to "take it one evolution at a time." If you look at all you have to do to overcome the obstacles, the goal may seem too far away. But McRaven says if you do your very best at that very moment, and take it one step at a time, then in six months you will have made it.[11]

Fortitude requires you to engage in constant positive self-talk. It requires an understanding that short-term goals will lead to long-term success. It is the understanding that it isn't how many times you get knocked down, but how many times you dust yourself off and get back up that counts.

While many principles reference external strength, fortitude is mostly internal strength. It takes perseverance, passion, and purpose. It is mental muscle that is developed through the discipline of staying positive and forging ahead. It is a necessary ingredient to winning fights and separates the ordinary from the great. Warriors with fortitude are difficult to beat. It's hard to beat someone who keeps getting back up. Fortitude is that internal strength required to never quit and never give up. It is a formidable principle.

NOTES

1. Joseph LeDoux, "Evolution of Human Emotion," *Progress and Brain Research* 195 (2012): 431–442; Jerome Popp, *Evolution's First Philosopher: John Dewey and the Continuity of Nature* (New York: SUNY Press, 2012).
2. Eric Zorn, "Without Failure, Jordan Would Be False Idol," *Chicago Tribune*, May 19, 1997, http://articles.chicagotribune.com/1997-05-19/news/9705190 096_1_nike-mere-rumor-driver-s-license.
3. Taylor et al., *Predictors of Success in Basic Underwater Demolition/SEAL (BUD/s) Training* (San Diego, CA: Naval Health Research Center, 2006).
4. Ranger Training Brigade Staff, *Ranger Handbook: SH 21-76* (Ft. Benning, GA: U.S. Army Infantry School, 2006).
5. Fred Pushies, *US Special Ops* (London: Voyageur Press, 2016).
6. Kenneth J. McAuliffe Jr., ed., *The Story of NUTS! Reply* (U.S. Army, 2012), https://www.army.mil/article/92856.
7. Peter Kreeft, *Back to Virtue*, Chapter 4: *Justice, Wisdom, Courage and Moderation: The Four Cardinal Virtues*, 59–70 (San Francisco, CA: Ignatius Press, 1986), 59–70.

8. Doreothea Frede, "Plato's Ethics: An Overview," *The Stanford Encyclopedia of Philosophy* (Winter Edition, 2016), https://plato.stanford.edu/entries/plato-ethics/.

9. Eve Light Honthaner, *Hollywood Drive: What It Takes to Break in, Hang in & Make It in the Entertainment Industry* (Abingdon-on-Thames, UK: Focal Press, 2013), 325.

10. William McRaven, *Make Your Bed: Little Things That Can Change Your Life . . . and Maybe the World* (New York: Grand Central Publishing, 2017).

11. Eames Yates, "A Navy SEAL Commander Explains How He Learned to Never Give Up," *Business Insider*, May 2, 2017, http://www.businessinsider.com/navy-seal-commander-explains-how-he-learned-never-give-up-william-mcraven-2017-4.

思想

リーダー 武蔵

STRIKING THOUGHTS

WHAT IS THE OBJECTIVE? What is the goal? These are two questions that must be answered when entering a fight. They are the two questions a Native American mentor drilled into my brain when teaching me how to tackle any problem.

Obviously, if the fight is unplanned the answers are simple and pre-answered. The goal is to survive and the objective to obtain the goal is to destroy or escape the enemy or opponent. In the broad sense the questions should be answered before the fight begins.

A fighter must at least decide during preparation what his answers are in order to establish a framework for his response to conflict. Are you more prepared to fight or escape? How have you prepared to meet the objective of winning during violence? Intelligence isn't so much as having all the right answers as asking the right questions. To win fights means to ask honest questions of your capabilities, situation, and goals.

Preparing for violent encounters means deciding how you will respond to violence and depends on many factors. But any fight on any scale requires going into the fight with an objective and a goal in mind that takes your resources and capabilities into consideration.

This illustrates the difference between these two questions. They are not the same thing. If a fight is planned, such as a battle or a sporting event, then the answers to these questions may initially be a bit broader in order to win. They are narrowed by preparation and even further narrowed through awareness when conflict is imminent.

A "goal" is achievement of an effort. It is a result. The goal is the ultimate desired outcome. It may seem obvious that the goal is to ultimately win. But a fighter must firmly decide to win and set it as a goal with a plan to achieve it. A fighter can't go through life or a fight by swinging blindly. No one can win on the street, in a ring, or at life without the focus of a goal.

The term "objective" can be a synonym of "goal," but is also best viewed in this context as the intended actions along the way to achieve the ultimate goal. The goal of course is the ultimate objective. But viewing it in this sense provides a framework of a long-term goal and short-term targets or objectives along the way that create a path to winning.

Mike Tyson said, "Everyone has a plan until they get punched in the mouth."[1] This is why principles are important. A real plan utilizes ancient principles that have survived 2,000 years of conflict. Principles take over when you get punched in the face and the typical fight plan begins to fall apart. Principles are foundational to winning and are solid rocks that will survive the storm. Beginning fighters become warriors by building character because winning principles arise from building honorable character.

MODERN WARRIORS

When researching this book, I sent a survey to a few fighters who ranged from amateurs to professional soldiers. Responses came from Special Forces Operators, marines, and other warriors.

I added the timing principle, since it was important to professionals and may not have been covered sufficiently under other principles. Timing is what a batter does in baseball. Upsetting timing is what a pitcher does in baseball. It is a difficult but important principle that is often overlooked.

Interviews with these professional fighters added the principle of fortitude. Historically, fortitude was an obvious principle of fighting, particularly when swords and battle-axes were in use. But today it seems to be in short supply. It needs a fresh look and prominent place among principles.

Maybe it was technology that made fighting cleaner from a distance. Maybe it was the protective behavior over our younger generation that all parents are guilty of today. Maybe it is political correctness that is rampant in society. Whatever the cause, the result is our youth may be losing the meaning of fortitude and can't appreciate a never-quit attitude in modern society. Reality is something our youth must grapple with in modern times. Life is not fair but we have to get used to it. The world doesn't care about our self-esteem. Our school systems may have eliminated winners and losers, but life hasn't. These are hard lessons. I added fortitude as a prominent twelfth principle in the hope that it hasn't been lost to antiquity.

Survey respondents consistently listed preparation in feedback as the first principle, in order of importance. It's an obvious first choice. Lethality was the second most important, which technically may be the most important principle as preparation is an inevitable first principle. All other principles seem to be vehicles to accomplish the ultimate goal of doing what is necessary to win. So a fighter that is lethal is a fighter that wins. The totalities of all the principles come together to make the fighter lethal, and lethality is what military operators attempt to achieve.

Fierceness, which is closely associated with lethality, was another top principle favored by professional warriors along with commitment. In fact, preparation, lethality, fierceness, and commitment were the top four principles that Special Forces operators felt were of prime importance to winning fights. After timing and fortitude were added, fortitude became popular among professional warriors who have reviewed these principles.

PERSPECTIVE

The world is a dangerous place. Distractions are increasing. Weapons are more deadly. Methods to inflict destruction are improving and our privacy is being diminished each day. Our attention is constantly being tugged in many directions and information availability is increasing at a rapid pace, which research shows doesn't necessarily improve our ability to make decisions.

Fighters have access to the best training methods and technology ever devised. Sports medicine and modern methods now create the best athletes mankind has ever known. But while techniques, methods, and application of technological advances change with time, principles remain the same.

It is the principles that haven't changed in 2,000 years that make the difference between a thug and a warrior. It is principles that determine who wins fights. Techniques are important, but they are flexible with time and adapt to change. Principled fighters are men of character who fight with honor.

Principles are under attack in modern society. Detractors say they are outdated. Focus is being lost in a technological society. Commitment is a principle that is fleeting. Discipline has been lost to short attention spans.

Political correctness threatens to turn principle on its head convincing the world that good is bad and bad is good. Wimps are being created over warriors. Modern society is a different environment for the warrior who is now a rare commodity. Principles are therefore more important now than ever before. We need principled people to protect freedom, combat crime, and even win the war of words as statesmen. How do we remain steadfast during such chaotic times and with so much opposition to principle?

Marcus Aurelius was a Roman emperor and an influential philosopher. He is attributed with saying, "When you wake up in the morning, tell yourself: the people I deal with today will be meddling, ungrateful, arrogant, dishonest, jealous and surly. They are like this because they can't tell good from evil. But I have seen the beauty of good, and the ugliness of evil."[2]

The quote is from his meditations and reflects his thoughts on what his father taught him about honor and humility. It is the same honor my father spoke about, and probably yours did as well. Honor and humility are things we should preserve.

The quote by Aurelius is a thought on how to keep one's sanity in an ever-changing world and succeed with inner peace. It is a challenge to rise above it all. We can't change the whole world but we can change ourselves and maybe impact our small corner of it.

Character and discipline must come before winning. If you build that first, winning will follow, as character isn't about how a fighter handles success. It's how a fighter handles failures.

Anyone who thinks they are going to build a martial arts or sports program without first building character and discipline believes a formalized program of study builds character. It doesn't.

Adversity and hard times doesn't necessarily develop character either. Adversity and challenges simply reveal character. These challenges then differentiate which fighter developed the necessary fortitude to win. But make no mistake, fortitude starts with character and discipline and is buoyed by honor. This is the warrior code derived from ancient wisdom.

STRENGTH

Fortis fortuna adiuvio (fortune favors the strong) is a Latin proverb that is so old it reflects spellings used by the same Romans who threw Christians to the lions. Its meaning is hotly debated by modern day fans of the *John Wick* franchise since Keanu Reeves portrayed the dark character with this phrase tattooed across his back. The essence of the proverb should have more clarity now. Its pagan origins seem to contrast the idea that, "the meek shall inherit the earth." But the strong are the meek. As discussed, the Greek term *praus* does not suggest weakness. It is simply disciplined strength. It is strength brought under control. Strength is channeled into great power. Only those with honorable character wield this power, and this is why character must first be developed in any fighter.

A warrior understands the contrast between these ideas of what it means to be strong. He trains his hands for war while remaining content to tend his garden. Those who understand these principles are prepared for realities we often wish did not exist.

In reality, the strong do win. Though we cheer for underdogs, they seldom win. They are underdogs for various reasons. Goliath usually wins. But developing character and utilizing time-honored principles allows fighters like the biblical David to emerge—fighters who are seemingly underdogs, but are truly strong. Goliath, bullies, and thugs do not have a chance against principled fighters who refuse to fight their opponents' fight. They fight their own fight.

If it were strength alone that was needed to win fights, we couldn't differentiate a warrior from a thug. Strength must be manifested not only by physical might but mental and spiritual might as well. Strength must be developed in every dimension.

These qualities coupled with humility enable warriors with strong character to aid the underdog and protect the weak. A warrior willing to deliver violence against evil is what secures peace.

Imperfect men and women have risen gallantly throughout the ages to face difficult tasks. But the principles perfected within them provided the tools forged by strength and perseverance that were necessary to complete the task. Principled fighters win.

IN THE DOJO

Fighters must be careful that their talent doesn't take them places their character cannot keep them. When entering a dojo a fighter thinks he wants to learn technique. What he really wants to leave with is principle.

There are few places left where this union of principle and character thrives. Military organizations, sports teams, law enforcement agencies, fire departments, rescue and EMS units are a few where brotherhood is understood and honor is valued.

Though I've visited some very fine dojos, gyms, and training schools, which are great places to learn to be a fighter, my dojo was small and personal, like many across the nation. Though I always trained with champions, the facilities were far from Olympic quality. The school seemed cramped. The smell of sweat lingered in the air. R&B music droned in the background. A dojo's value is measured by the principles you learn, not by the size of the building.

Your fellow fighters became your trusted friends. When you become black belts together you are brothers. Mine come from every creed, religion, and culture. The bond is forged through years of sweat, thousands of punches, hundreds of fights, countless bruises, and occasional blood. A black belt isn't something you wear, it is something you become. Common warrior principles create a common bond.

Wherever you train, from backyards to gymnasiums, seek not only to learn technique to deal with others. Seek principle to deal with yourself and you will find you win fights bigger than yourself. Your life will then be regulated by principle rather than rules. There is nothing that brings people together more than struggling for something worthwhile or something greater than themselves.

Lastly, fighters must keep each other accountable. I recall a young brown belt in his late twenties trying to impress a visiting sensei who was in his mid-sixties. The young fighter came very hard at the sensei during sparring. The elderly fighter had been a full contact champion and had to strike the young brown belt much harder than he probably wished and naturally was on the receiving end of some bruises himself. Brown belts tend to be the most vicious fighters as they are on the verge of becoming black belts and lack discipline over the skills they've learned. They also feel they have something to prove.

After a small amount of blood was spilled, one of our newer black belts put his arm around the young brown belt and took him to the side. He whispered politely to the young fighter. I later learned that this young black belt had quietly admonished the brown belt that attempting to go full contact with a guest and three times his age was disrespectful. The admonishment had less sting coming from a younger black belt who was one of the brown belt's peers rather than coming from one of us older black belts. Seeing the younger black belt lead provides hope for our future.

The young brown belt was held accountable in a polite manner by fellow fighters. He apologized to the sensei, who actually spent extra time with the young man. He learned his lesson and it cost him only a few drops of blood. He later became a black belt and a leader able to humbly hold other fighters accountable to honor as well.

The point is, there is a brotherhood among fighters. We should politely hold each other accountable to that honor and to warrior principles.

PARTING PRINCIPLES

When a fighter spends thousands of hours in a martial arts discipline, it is difficult for that discipline not to manifest itself in all areas of the fighter's life. This is why following these ancient principles is important, as understanding them will impact all areas of life.

The evil minority makes the peaceful majority irrelevant if peaceful men do nothing. These principles provide the arms to combat this complacency and allow you to become what you wish to be instead of what has happened to you. Be one of the few who feel the rain rather than simply getting wet.

Applying time-honored principles requires mental, spiritual, and physical discipline. Remember that thought occurs before action and nothing happens without a thought. There is a Chinese proverb sometimes attributed to Lao Tzu that, "Thoughts become words, words become actions, actions become habits, habits become character and character becomes one's destiny."

Times change and techniques adapt. But principles are everlasting. That's why principles win fights.

Notes

1. Mike Berardino, "Mike Tyson explains one of his most famous quotes," *Sun Sentinel*, November 9, 2012.
2. Marcus Aurelius, *Meditations,* translated by Gregory Hays (New York: Modern Library Classics, 2003), II, 1.

SECTION 2: PARTING PRINCIPLES

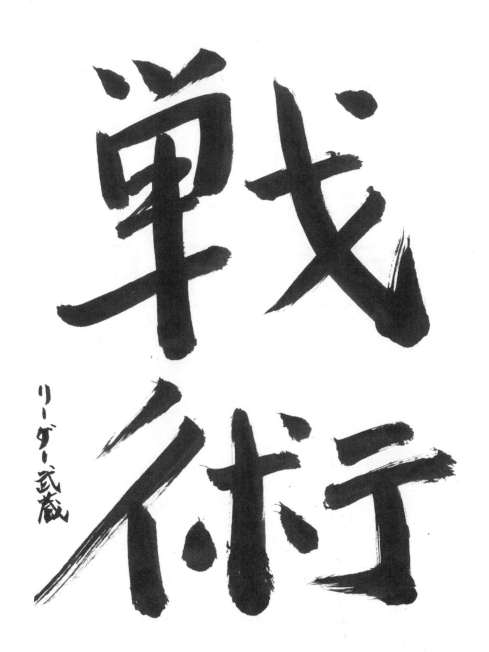

戦術

リーダー武蔵

FIGHTING WITH
TACTICS

WHILE STRATEGY and principles are broad goals, tactics are methods for accomplishing those goals. Every principle has tactical applications. Sun Tzu opined 2,000 years ago that strategy without tactics is the slowest route to victory and tactics without strategy is the noise before defeat.[1] This is why tactics must be understood along with principled strategy.

A fighter must bridge principles with actual methods that employ each principle at the tactical level. Here are some brief approaches to bridging strategy and tactics for each principle. There are many others, but this is a basic start to understanding the foundational connection between principles and strategy and how they are interconnected.

PREPARATION

The principle of preparation requires a decision regarding what you will do when faced with conflict. You must decide in advance and prepare in some manner. If the fighter is a competitor, then he must know every aspect of the competitive arena. There are rules that must be prepared, the opponents he will face should be known, and even the size of the area of combat must be studied. The fighter must train his mind and body for the event.

If the person has a goal of self-defense then there are many classes he or she can attend. Preparing to study martial arts requires understanding the level of interest and involvement the fighter wishes to invest. Preparing can begin in several ways and with classes such as hard styles, soft styles, classical approaches, or simply physical development gyms. Preparation involves many levels, from simple awareness to physical fitness conditioning or more advanced training, and should keep the interest of the practitioner.

Some people have little time to invest. Learning a martial art or going to the gym to work out every week doesn't fit their schedule. These individuals still must prepare for violent encounters or they will be the prey of predators. Preparation may involve different levels of investment for these folks, but it still must occur. They may wish to learn how to use weapons and certainly must plan their travels accordingly to avoid dangerous areas. Even trained fighters must prepare at this level by planning where they go and how they will react if violence greets them.

The point is to prepare on some level and then plan in advance as to how to apply this preparation. Deciding how you will react to violent encounters removes much of the fear of such encounters.

Businesses and nations have a whole different level of preparation. But on a tactical level they too must prepare a method to overcome challenges in their business or against enemies of the state. Tactical application of the principle depends on the scale of exposure that spans varying levels of investment and the scope of exposure ranging from individuals to nations. Decision models based on scenarios businesses or nations face on a broad scale should be incorporated into policy then tested and updated on a regular basis as threats change.

"What if" questions are a good way to start preparing on any level. What if a mugger faces you? What if multiple attackers appear? What if a weapon is produced? Reviewing potential scenarios and deciding on a course of action in advance is valuable to the tactical approach toward preparation. Anticipating encounters increases the level of preparedness. Mental and physical preparation on any level is vital.

AWARENESS

Knowing violence can occur and anticipating it is most of the battle. Keeping a 360-degree awareness of surroundings is important. This is an era of technology, which demands our attention. Those who wish to be aware of their surroundings cannot get sucked into their technology.

On a tactical level, fighters must look and anticipate. Sizing up situations is an instinct. People know when something isn't quite right or is out of place. To know what is normal in your surroundings and become very suspicious when patterns are broken is the tactical application of being aware. Again, awareness is more than being alert. Awareness is placing suspicions and broken patterns into context.

Putting away cell phones and looking around is the simplest way to increase awareness. Avoiding dangerous situations is a practical tactic. Seeing and knowing are symbiotic tactical applications of the principle of awareness.

Having a plan of escape or attack in any given situation places the fighter at a tactical advantage. If preparation has given the fighter the tools to win a possible engagement then awareness is the last line of defense to avoid the necessity of implementing this preparation. But in the event violence cannot be avoided, awareness robs the attacker of the element of surprise. Awareness counters the tactical advantage typically given to a predator.

Violence seldom occurs suddenly. There is often a build-up and a chance for de-escalation or escape. A fight occurs when awareness, avoidance, and de-escalation fail. Awareness is more an attitude than a skill. To be alert is not the same as being paranoid. Tactically, the idea is to remain alert and aware of the input provided by the surroundings.

COMMITMENT

During college, a friend of mine taught judo. He was an exchange student from Japan. Some other martial artists and I were taking a break from learning some judo throws and engaged in some striking skill practice.

We were demonstrating our methods of striking and delivered a snapping kick to the groin. The kick was focused on the groin. My Japanese friend said we were doing it all wrong. We were not committing fully to the action by simply focusing a kick to the groin only on the groin itself.

If we were fully committed to kicking someone between the legs and doing damage, we should not aim at the groin. We should aim for the chin. "If kicking groin, do not aim at groin. Aim at chin," he said in broken English.

He did this while motioning with his hands that we should visualize attempting to kick through the groin and up through the opponent's whole body to reach the chin. That was the greatest lesson I ever had regarding commitment to an action.

On a tactical level, commitment is a sense of certainty. It is being decisive and following a course of action. The tactical method to accomplish the principle of commitment is to make a decision in an unwavering fashion and acting on the decision with vigor. It is the same process you follow when jumping off a cliff to dive into the water below. At some point, you have to jump. One foot cannot be on the cliff and one foot off the cliff. You have to fully commit.

The Samurai applied this principle to every aspect of their life. We should as well. Full commitment has benefit in tactical application whether you are fully committing to a job, a marriage, a task, or a fight. If you leap into the task at hand, there is complete focus.

There must be no uncertainty. Once you have committed to an action in a decisive manner uncertainty will diminish. Tactically, the whole focus should then be on that action.

LETHALITY

Ruthless vigor is a good way to describe this principle in a tactical sense. Being ruthless is a way to win a fight. The practical tactical application of lethality in civil society requires varying degrees of aggression. There can only be enough force to repel the attack. This is why many law enforcement agencies have a caveat of scaled aggression when applying this principle. This is the reason the principle isn't simply being ruthless but having the potential to be lethal. So the caveat is to use just enough force to repel the attack.

But to be clear, the common denominator regardless of the level of aggression needed to repel an attack is that there must be the potential to take that aggression as far as tactically required to win the fight. Predators don't want to fight in general. They want to win. If they size up their victim and determine the victim will not be an easy target then the chances of a fight diminish. This means the intended victim must appear to have this quality of lethality. A fighter must be willing to do what is necessary to survive and win.

Firearms instructors will tell students in concealed carry classes that if they are not willing to kill another person who is threatening their life, then they should not carry a gun. They are simply bringing a weapon to a fight they are not willing to win, giving the attacker the advantage and possibly even giving the attacker a gun to do the job. The gun is not what makes the person carrying it lethal. It is the willingness to use the gun that makes the person lethal.

So on a tactical level this term of lethality must be understood in application. If understood, then more law enforcement agencies will accept the principle. When simply framed as brutality, the principle seems uncivil. Ruthlessness itself may not be required to win the fight. But the fighter must be willing to be ruthless if necessary. That is being lethal.

Sometimes just pulling a weapon can repel an attack. No further action is required. That is stopping the force at the level required to repel the attack. But the principle of lethality means that on a tactical level you are willing to do whatever is necessary to save your life. It's that simple.

If you are willing to go to whatever extreme is necessary to win, you are lethal. You don't necessarily have to unleash that lethality. You do not have to actually be ruthless, uncaring, unfeeling, or brutal. But you must be willing to exert those aspects if it becomes tactically necessary.

This is the tactical application of lethality. Being willing to do whatever it takes to win is being lethal. The level of lethality is a tactical component.

EFFICIENCY

A shotgun is a more efficient means of repelling multiple attackers than a pellet gun. It is fast, powerful, and requires less effort with limited chances of getting hurt if you have enough warning that multiple attackers are coming for you.

The tactical point is using what will do the best job in any given situation. Don't use a pellet gun if a shotgun will work better. Attack if you know you are going to be attacked anyway to end conflict quickly. Retreat if you face stronger opposition and are sure to be defeated if you do not retreat. Decide what action will work best in the shortest amount of time.

When faced with a mugger, it is sometimes best to turn and run in the opposite direction. That is tactical efficiency. It is the fastest and easiest way to victory. You have avoided a fight or ended the fight by the path of least resistance.

Efficiency is the use of minimum effort to achieve maximum results. The strategy of efficiency relates to effectiveness as well. The two are often confused.

Effectiveness is different from efficiency. A shotgun blast will effectively kill an ant. But it is terribly inefficient. You must load the gun and damage surrounding surfaces, not to mention it is overkill. A simple flick of a finger would be fast with less effort. A shotgun is effective in killing an ant. A flick of the finger is efficient.

If your tactical application is both efficient and effective then you have found the perfect combination. Lt. Col. Jeff Cooper said the goal of the tactition is to ensure the fight isn't fair.[2] It is a quote pointed out earlier and it can't be said enough. This embodies the tactical concept of efficiency. Use whatever is best suited to get the job done and requires the most economical use of force to accomplish the task. Marines have a saying that the only unfair fight is the one you lose.

Efficiency is the relationship between the means and the end. If the method is efficient, then no more means are employed to accomplish the end. There is this nice balance. If a method is inefficient, then the end could have been achieved by less means or the means employed produced more than the desired result.[3]

DISCIPLINE

Marine Major General James Mattis once said, "Be polite, be professional, but have a plan to kill everybody you meet."[4] It was one of the rules he gave his marines deployed to Iraq. He also famously said, "I come in peace. I didn't bring artillery. But I'm pleading with you, with tears in my eyes; If you (mess) with me, I'll kill you all." This was the message he sent to Iraqi leaders following the invasion. He commanded a deadly fighting force. He expressed his willingness to use that force. But he was disciplined in when to use force.

Being calm and in full control of your actions provides you a tactical advantage. Causing the opposition to lose their cool can be advantageous, as they will make mistakes. Being in control of yourself is an important tactical advantage and requires discipline and focus.

A marine firearms instructor informed his students that anything worth shooting was worth shooting twice. Ammunition is cheap. Life is expensive.

This correlated with discipline one day when a Special Forces operator accidently shot his sergeant during a training exercise. The young soldier was chastised for his lack of discipline when he visited the recovering sergeant in the hospital. The sergeant said he had taught the young man to put two rounds into anything he shot. The sergeant received only one wound and had trained his men to fire two rounds into every target. He expected better discipline out of his men, even when they accidentally shot him.

Tactical discipline is being courteous but not necessarily friendly. Be nice but not completely trusting. It is being nervous but not letting them see you sweat. Take deep breaths and remain calm under fire. Discipline has all of these elements and is a tactical challenge. It is the essence of what General Mattis expressed in his colorful quotes.

We've discussed that those who remain calm under fire share certain traits. They see obstacles as an opportunity, focus on improving whatever situation they are in regardless of how bad the situation becomes, and remain committed by never giving up. Accomplishing all of this while maintaining composure is tactical discipline.

These tactical traits are important and must be clearly understood. They are worth listing:[5,6]

1. Uncertainty must be viewed as an opportunity.
2. Always focus on improving your situation.
3. Never quit.

Disciplined fighters are not impulsive. They are not guided by first impressions. This is how an experienced fighter sometimes lures a novice fighter. He may feign an attack to get a young fighter to commit to an action. The experienced fighter is then ready to counter after drawing his opponent into his trap. This is maintaining fight discipline.

Recognizing when and when not to act along with being calm during action so as not to be impulsive is not always natural. Discipline must be cultivated. Experience and practice help develop discipline. Cool-headed action develops under the influence of discipline, as cool-headedness cannot exist without self-control.

Chesty Puller was a Marine Corps lieutenant general who fought in World War II and the Korean conflict. He is the most decorated marine in U.S. history. He is admired by his friends and feared by his enemies. To this day, marines at Parris Island will end their day or do one more push-up acknowledging Chesty. Upon seeing a flamethrower demonstration for the first time he asked where the bayonet was.

But his most famous demonstration of calm discipline under fire putting all these traits to action was when the enemy had his men surrounded. Chesty said, "We've been looking for the enemy for some time now. We've finally found him. We're surrounded. That simplifies our problem of getting to these people and killing them."[7]

Being calm during stress is a critical tactical element. It allows for assessing danger, its nature, and how to manage it. Once the cause of fear is defined it ceases to exist to a certain extent, as the unknown is usually the greatest fear. The bottom line is that tactical discipline is the ability to keep a cool head, and it is an important principle.

POWER

Though the overarching principle is power, speed is the driving force of power at the tactical level. Actually, the principle could very well be speed and really is speed in many texts on war. But power is expressed as mass multiplied by speed and provides a much broader term. Therefore, speed is understood as the critical element of power. So for the record, speed is an essential tactical property of power. But power incorporates all the necessary elements and is more foundational to a fight. Speed is a tactic to accomplish power.

A quick look at power versus force will help to understand this relationship. The technical aspects are interesting. Force is the interaction of two objects moved by a push or a pull, so force occurs over a distance between objects. The amount of work is force applied over a distance.

Power is the rate at which work is expressed. If force is the distance of work, power is the time rate of work. Power is how quickly the work is done. Now you see the close relationship.[8]

A small amount of quickly expressed force generates a great deal of power. It's why snatching a rope tied to a load will move it but gradually pulling might not generate enough power to move it.

Martial artists develop power by training their muscles to coordinate into motions kinesiology refers to as kinetic linking. The mystics call it *ki*, which in the Kanji Japanese symbol is essentially steam coming from rice, which describes energy.[9]

Training helps to focus energy. Wasted motion generates less power. Putting your hips into a throw or throwing the whole body into a punch are examples. This is how Bruce Lee accomplished his amazing 1 inch punch: through speed and kinetic linking.

While raw strength does have a tactical advantage in winning a fight, it is explosiveness of action and efficient delivery of force that generates power. The idea in winning a fight is to transfer as much destructive power as possible to the opponent. But again, the difference between a push and a strike is the amount of time it takes to deliver them. As time decreases, the push becomes a strike, which emphasizes again the importance of speed to power.

Recall the physics behind power; that speed increases mass. On the tactical level it is fine to lift weights to increase a fighters' strength. But a punch isn't the same as a bench press. If you need strength to push the opponent, this type of strength is helpful. But the power of a punch is increased with speed as this increases its energy.

Tactical application of power requires training and understanding how to apply the principles. It is only through preparation that maximum tactical advantage can be attained through power. Most important, this tactical advantage isn't limited to size. Power is as much about explosiveness and speed as it is about raw strength or force alone.

Focus

While there are mental and physical aspects to the principle of focus it is a tactical challenge to merge the two concepts. Research has shown that keeping the eyes steady without blinking slows the perception of time. Experiencing a disaster seems to slow time. Many situations where intense focus is involved seem to slow time.[10]

Time has subjective and objective components, which are altered by focus.

Focus is sometimes about concentration and trained responses. Beginning martial artists learn step-by-step processes. Each movement must be understood, analyzed, and executed. Nothing is yet automatic. Neural imaging in scientific research has revealed that beginners mostly utilize the prefrontal cortex of the brain, which is responsible for conscious concentration, when learning moves.

More experienced martial artists utilize the basal ganglia. This area of the brain is responsible for muscle memory, the physical sense of touch, and feeling sensations through the skin by touch. The more experienced fighter therefore is able to integrate complex combinations more efficiently in a way that is practically impossible for the beginner. Accessing different areas of the brain to execute movements and undergo training alters the very structure of the brain.[11]

Beginning fighters must focus on step-by-step learning. Practice does make perfect, as concentration begins to develop a different level of focus and execution. Movements and actions become hardwired into the brain.

The mental focus that seems to slow time and the physical focus that places action into muscle memory have tactical utility. Merging these two concepts with the concept of commitment allows a martial artist to break many bricks. The martial artist focuses energy on a point and concentrates on striking through the target, not simply at it. In a fight these movements are much faster and automatic due to training.

Tactically, focus is concentrating energy on what to hit or action to take. This focus can be trained and science is learning that even subjective perception of time changes with focus. Focus helps apply the other principles.

FIERCENESS

If lethality is the willingness to be as lethal as necessary to win, ferocity is the expression of lethality in terms of aggressiveness and needed brutality. Tactical operations succeed mostly through three core elements:

1. Speed
2. Surprise
3. Violent Action

Ferocity is aggressive violent action. You can see how these principles begin to intertwine when you understand that a fighter must be disciplined, humble, and respectful while training in a dojo in order to learn to be an effective warrior. Hostility is an impediment to learning.

But if met in an alley by an attacker, a humble presence will not make an effective warrior that wins the fight. This is the paradox of martial arts. A warrior must possess both humbleness and ferocity to succeed. Aristotle referred to courage as a balance between cowardice and rashness.[12] Being overly meek is cowardly. Being overly fierce results in rage. Discipline balances the two. But it isn't a compromise between them. There is a tactical difference.

A knight in medieval times had a code of chivalry. He was to be fierce to the maximal degree when necessary to win a battle. But he was to be meek to the maximal degree when not in battle. Aristotle felt the virtuous person was continually seeking the correct degree on the scale of the extremes in each situation.

In this sense, it takes courage for the warrior to be meek when necessary as much as it is being ferocious when necessary. Being able to exert a great deal of violence from a peaceful person are not mutually exclusive concepts. This is the tactical application of ferocity and demonstrates the many paradoxes that exist among the principles.

The fighter must be able to apply the level of aggressiveness necessary to win the engagement. But he must also understand there is a scale and that it takes courage to find the right level.

Being able to exert violence is not in opposition to peace but actually a necessary component of ensuring peace. Protecting loved ones is an act of love as you are willing to defend them. Standing up to evil requires willingness to exert violence.

Tactical fierceness is to exhibit extreme violence. It is flipping a mental switch and being the most aggressive fighter.

SURPRISE

Surprise is one of the most important tactical elements in winning fights. The problem is that surprise is often sacrificed to the initial aggressor. But even in a self-defense posture, surprise is a powerful tactical tool as unexpected actions exert this principle.

Examine any list of principles of war throughout history or from any nation's military science manual and surprise is included. Striking an opponent in a manner for which he is unprepared shifts the balance of power. Surprising actions leverage success out of proportion to the actual expended effort.

Sun Tzu wrote the earliest principles of war and suggested surprise could come in many forms. Location, timing, and force of response are just some of the unexpected forms of surprise. Sun Tzu said that all warfare was based on deception and deception is a powerful tool. Deception is surprise.

To tactically create surprise requires the fighter to strike before the opponent is ready for the strike. That is surprise on a tactical level.

Even if the opponent is prepared for the attack, changing the method of attack for which the opponent is unprepared can create surprise. Again, deploying an attack, strike, or action that the opponent does not anticipate creates surprise. Your opponent may be ready to fight, but he may be ready for the wrong fight.

One of the earliest examples of this tactic involved the ancient Greeks. Typically, the ancient soldier carried his shield in his left hand and his spear in his right. This made the right wing of a group of soldiers vulnerable. To compensate, military leaders would generally put their best soldiers on the right wing of the group. The right wing then became the strongest part of the force.

Naturally, battles at the time were usually decided by which army was able to have its own right wing quickly defeat the other side's weaker left wing. Then turn in a flanking maneuver over the defeated left wing to attack the right wing of their enemy, which would now be fighting soldiers in front of them and to their left flank.

In 371 BCE, Theban general Epaminondas knew the Spartans would use this tactic with their strongest men on the right. So he developed an unexpected tactic to surprise the Spartans. He over-strengthened the left wing of his own force. Then he advanced toward the Spartans in an oblique line rather than head-on.[13]

The intent was for his strong Theban left wing to come into contact with the Spartan right wing first before his now weaker Theban right wing was even engaged in battle. Though he reversed the usual tactic, he still protected his weaker right wing by attacking at an angle so that it was not engaged until most of the stronger soldiers were weakened on the other side. Although Epaminondas was outnumbered and had inferior forces, he won the conflict.

TIMING

Hitting the objective at the right moment is the tactical application of timing. In execution, timing is understanding when to strike, how to strike, where to strike, and what to strike. In a broader sense, it may even be who to strike, though tactically, timing is getting to the right target at the exact moment that opportunity provides the best opening.

Timing is not only when to strike but when to retreat, speak, or go to the ground. It may also be upsetting the timing of your opponent. We've discussed ancient Samurai who showed up late to a fight or utilized other techniques simply to disrupt the timing of an enemy. Much of this has to do with reaction time.

Reaction time is a measure of how one responds to stimulus. The average reaction time in humans is 0.25 seconds to visual stimuli, 0.17 for audio, and 0.15 for touch.[14] Research has shown that practicing an activity shortens reaction time, which may be due to the tactical preparation of hardwiring coordinated movements into the brain.[15]

Research also suggests muscle strength may decrease the reaction time of the muscle as well, as men average a reaction time a fraction faster than women.[16] Therefore, strength and experience are contributing factors that lower reaction time. The lower the reaction time the more time a fighter has to execute proper timing.

FORTITUDE

Always see yourself winning. Always visualize yourself continuing to fight. A proper mental attitude is vital to tactically applying fortitude.

Nick Vujicic was born without arms and legs, yet he is a happy person who is a motivational speaker. He plays sports, travels, is married, and has children. He is a classic example of how positive mental attitude translates into never giving up.[17]

Navy Seal training also exemplifies that a strong mental attitude is vital to winning. With a 70 percent dropout rate, only those with a forged mental fortitude complete the training.[18] Seals understand that most of fortitude is mental. Seals refuse to listen to that inner voice that urges them to quit. Physical pain is temporary, but the pain of quitting lasts longer.

The first step in applying fortitude is mental discipline. Seals take a slow deep breath to calm themselves. Ancient warriors engaged in meditation techniques.

The next step is to have a goal. Even short-term goals are useful. In fact, Seal trainees who had short-term goals were less likely to quit than those who had no goals or worried about what was going to happen in the long term. The goal may be as simple as not quitting for at least the next hour. Goal setting helps us to take things one step at a time. Confucius said, "The man who moves mountains begins by carrying small stones."[19]

Mental focus is another step toward developing mental toughness. As noted previously, mental visualization can improve performance. Positive words are an important element. Self-talk should always be positive, not negative.

Fighters should not allow emotions to get the best of them or to cloud judgment. Mentally tough people have learned how to stay calm during heated adversity. Rolling with the punches is a good analogy. Find a source of motivation, relax, and be flexible enough to adapt to changing situations. This resiliency will help to bring mental toughness to a fight.

There is an old proverb regarding the transient nature of anything good or bad. A Persian ruler asked wise men for a quote that would be true in all situations. After consultation they concluded with the words, "This too shall pass."[20]

Listen to motivational speakers. Surround yourself with positive quotes. Be a reader with a book constantly nearby. Allow all your senses to be engulfed by positive messages and allow positive words to be a constant part of your vocabulary. You become what you constantly read. What you constantly speak becomes reality.

Tactical application of fortitude is vital in a society that increasingly does not appreciate delayed gratification or quits when the least amount of adversity arises. Mental toughness is necessary to persevere when quitting seems to be the only option.

Tactical Review

Unlike principles, tactics change according to the situation. For example, winning a fight by avoiding confrontation is a great principle that arises out of preparation and awareness. A tactic to execute this principle would be to run away from a robber.

But on the playground a bully might pursue you, or in the case of a robber, you may have a loved one to protect. The tactic of running might not be the best option in these scenarios. Tactics may apply principles differently depending on the situation.

There is a daily barrage of messages from coworkers, politicians, religious leaders, media, and a multitude of other sources. There is a constant marketplace competing for ideas and demanding your attention. This turbulence creates noise that is constant static in our lives. Values seem to change. Morals seem to be flexible with time. Our thoughts are continually challenged each day.

What is needed are individuals who apply time-honored principles that do not change with time. Principles examine the bigger picture of life, providing needed stability in a sea of turbulent thought.

Tactics apply these principles. Tactics can be adapted to the situation, but the principles never change.

NOTES

1. Sun Tzu, *The Art of War and Other Classics of Eastern Thought* (New York: Barnes & Noble, 2013).

2. Jeff Cooper, *Principles of Personal Defense* (Boulder, CO: Paladin Press, 2006).

3. Stephen Palmer, "Definitions of Efficiency," *British Medical Journal* 318 (1999): 1136.

4. Madeline Conway, "9 Unforgettable Quotes by James Mattis" *Politico* (December 1, 2016), http://www.politico.com/blogs/donald-trump-administra tion/2016/12/james-mattis-quotes-232097.

5. Vishnu Virtues, "6 Qualities of People Who Never Quit," *Addicted 2 Success Blog*, n.d., https://addicted2success.com/success-advice/6-qualities-of-people -who-never-quit/.

6. Carolyn Gregoire, "The 9 Essential Habits of Mentally Strong People," *Huffingtonpost Blog* (February 18, 2014), http://www.huffingtonpost.com/2014 /02/18/the-9-essential-qualitie_n_4760403.html.

7. Ben Thompson, "Chesty Puller," *The Badass of the Week Blog*, n.d., http:// www.badassoftheweek.com/puller.html.

8. Karin Nice, "How Force, Power, Torque and Energy Work," *Howstuffworks .com*, n.d., http://auto.howstuffworks.com/auto-parts/towing/towing-capacity /information/fpte.htm.

9. Dave Lowry, *Sword and Brush: The Spirit of the Martial Arts* (Boulder, CO: Shambhala Publications, 1995).

10. David Eagleman, "Human Time Perception and Its Illusions," *Current Opinion in Neurobiology* 18 (2008): 131–136.

11. Roberts et al., "Individual Differences in Expert Motor Coordination Associated with White Matter Microstructure in the Cerebellum," *Cerebral Cortex* 23 (2013): 2282–2292.

12. Aristotle, "Nicomachean Ethics," W. D. Ross, trans., Internet Classics Archive, Massachusetts Institute of Technology, n.d., http://classics.mit.edu/Aristotle /nicomachaen.html.

13. Mark Cartwright, "Greek Warfare," *Ancient History Encyclopedia*, last modified May 17, 2013, http://www.ancient.eu/Greek_Warfare/.

14. Marsha Matyas, "Neural Networks," *APS Education* (2002), https://webcache .googleusercontent.com/search?q=cache:v-QnxHadA1wJ:https://www.lifescitrc .org/download.cfm%3FsubmissionID%3D6968+&cd=21&hl=en&ct=clnk&gl =us&client=safari.

15. Haugen Tonnessen and Shalfawi, "Reaction Time Aspects of Elite Sprinters in Athletic World Championships," *Journal of Strength & Conditioning Research* 27 (2013): 885–892.

16. Stephen Lord, Gideon Caplan, and John Ward, "Balance, Reaction Time and Muscle Strength in Exercising and Nonexercising Older Women: A Pilot Study," *Archives of Physical Medicine and Rehabilitation* 74 (1993): 837–839; A. Jain et al., "A Comparative Study of Visual and Auditory Reaction Times on the Basis of Gender and Physical Activity Levels of Medical First Year Students," *International Journal of Applied Basic Medical Research* 5 (2015): 124–127.

17. "Nick Vujicic," Wikipedia, last modified June 18, 2017, https://en.wikipedia.org/wiki/Nick_Vujicic.

18. James Dao, "Heavy Toll in Afghan Fight for Navy's Proud Elite," *New York Times*, July 9, 2005, http://www.nytimes.com/2005/07/09/us/heavy-toll-in-afghan-fight-for-navys-proud-elite.html.

19. Chinese Language Beta, "Confucius Quote," Stackexchange.com, https://chinese.stackexchange.com/questions/12115/confucius-quote-whats-the-original.

20. "This Too Shall Pass," Wikipedia, last modified May 5, 2017, https://en.wikipedia.org/wiki/This_too_shall_pass.

名誉

リーダー武蔵

FIGHTING WITH
HONOR

ANY BOOK ABOUT winning fights would be incomplete without a chapter on honor. But these days it might not be self-evident as the meaning of honor has faded and has been distorted. My father used the word "honor" more than any other word when he was teaching me about growing into manhood. Today he would be considered from the "old school" of thought. He came from an era when a man's word was his bond. If my father shook your hand on a deal it was better than any signature on a contract. He was respected. Honor had meaning. It had meaning to his entire generation. So during my life I sought out men of honor who shared this philosophy, as sadly honor seems to be less important with each generation.

Honor is a symbol of distinction. It is a good name the public holds in high esteem. An honorable person is respectful and in turn is shown respect. An honorable person earns this respect by having a keen sense of ethical conduct.

Merited honor is something that separates a warrior from a thug. The concept of "no honor among thieves" captures the observations of King Solomon: "The soul of the wicked desireth evil: his neighbor findeth no favour in his eyes."[1]

Honor is something a fighter must possess to become a true warrior.

THE WARRIOR CODE

Honor was one of the eight Samurai codes of virtue. It was the code of the Bushido.[2] Though *Bushido* means "the way of the warrior" and focuses much on fighting and war, it was equally concerned with nonmartial behavior. This code stressed values of loyalty and honor to family and country, which were valued in fighters. This is the type of honor that separates a thug or predator from a professional warrior or civilized person. Both thug and warrior have the ability to inflict violence. But only the warrior engages in violence for an honorable purpose.

Within the warrior code it was written that the Samurai were to have a vivid consciousness of personal dignity and worth. Samurai exhibited true patience, bearing the unbearable in order to avoid being seen as short-tempered. They did not take offense to a minor provocation, as this would bring disgrace to their character. They either fought with all their might to destroy an enemy or they didn't fight at all if the fight had no merit. Honor had everything to do with the nature of conflict. It had everything to do with the fight. Honor put the fight into context.

The Samurai were feared in large part because of this nonmartial character trait. They were disciplined enough not to fight over a minor offense. But if they did fight, they fought with 100 percent ferocity and commitment as their honor and reputation were at stake. The offender would not walk away from a fight with a Samurai who was fighting due to this deeply ingrained value. Fighting simply for the sake of fighting doesn't make a warrior. There are things that bring honor or shame to a warrior and fighting with purpose is one of them.

Fighting unjustly or for no reason is unconscionable in the view of ancient warriors. Fighting without purpose or a cause greater than oneself brings shame. There must be some code of ethics guiding a fighter or the fight is simply shameful. It is this code of ethics that makes the fighter an honorable warrior. The fight has purpose, fighting against a malevolent force within the bounds of these ethics.

The exception was when both warriors agreed to test their skills. Fighting for sport was not unheard of in ancient civilizations. Warriors continue this desire to test their skills today and still adhere to honorable ethics.

Shameful fights are senseless arguments over minor provocation, verbal conflicts that escalate, or a bully picking a fight with an innocent victim. It takes men of honor to take a stand against shameless violence or repel evil intent.[3]

Only those with honor who are skilled in violence can defeat evil. Certainly, defeating evil may require barbarous actions by a warrior. But fighting for a noble purpose and behaving according to a code of honor prevents these warriors from becoming barbarians themselves. It can actually be a tricky construct.

Warriors are not sociopaths. Honor within the warrior code and fighting for a purpose separates a warrior engaging in warfare from a serial killer. Warriors respect values. Sociopaths do not.

In this view, not all fighters are warriors. Warriors are men of honor.

Confucius said that the superior man seeks what is right. The inferior man seeks what is profitable.[4] Therefore, honor is about the internal motivation of the warrior seeking what is right and just.

This is illustrated in Greek mythology. Achilles and Hector were contrasting heroes found in *The Iliad*, which was written around 720 BCE. Achilles led the Greek army and Hector commanded the Trojans.

Both were great warriors and heroes of their people. But their motivation separated them. Fame and fortune motivated Achilles, who fought for personal gain. He was moved by his own emotions and revenge.

Hector saw his role as defender of Troy. He was motivated by what was best for his country and his people. He held deep devotion for his family. Even after battle he permitted the enemy to care for their injured. Hector has been viewed as the more honorable of the two.

Hector killed Achilles's cousin Patroclus in battle. Patroclus fought secretly using Achilles's armor and Hector mistook him for Achilles. Achilles then sought out Hector for revenge.[5]

There are many complexities in ancient mythology. Achilles was a hero motivated by his own desires and eventually killed by an arrow shot into his heel. (This is the origin of "Achilles heel," which refers to someone's weak point.)

Hector was guided by rational thought, honor, and integrity. He could control his emotions though Achilles overpowered him. The story illustrates the difference between a fighter who acts out of anger, allowing emotions to control his actions, rather than out of a sense of honor and wisdom. Honor is what differentiates the mere fighter from a fighter who is a warrior. The seventeenth-century writer Francois de La Rochefoucauld wrote that, "The glory of great men must always be measured against the means they have used to acquire it."[6]

In 1900, Inazo Nitobe wrote *Bushido: The Soul of Japan*. It was a book of Japanese culture and one of the first books on Samurai ethics written for Western readers. This is the first Western source of the Eight Virtues of Bushido, which are:

1. Honor

   A sense of high ethical conduct. One's word is a guarantee. The warrior has credibility because he gives his word then lives up to it. Respect is shown to other people and is reflected in the warrior's actions. Honor is rooted in personal dignity.

2. Righteousness (Rectitude - Justice)

   The exhibition of honesty in dealing with others. As a theological concept, it is an attribute denoting that a person's actions are justified and that he or she leads a life that is pleasing to God. This was one of the highest virtues, which provided the Samurai the power to decide on a course of action without wavering. When you think about it, if there is no higher power, then what is the value of a moral code?

3. Courage

   A willingness to face uncertainty and danger and choosing to act appropriately when confronted with opposition. Samurai warriors were known for bravery but possessing courage is more than being brave. Courage must be exercised for the cause of righteousness and justice. To be courageous, one will do what is right regardless of the circumstances

4. Compassion (Benevolence)

   Warriors' power is used for good. They are kind to others and show mercy. A Samurai had great power and it was expected that someone with such power exhibited qualities of benevolence and mercy. Knowing when not to use power is as important as knowing when to exert it.

5. Respect (Politeness)

This addresses the respect shown to warriors and the deference they show others. Warriors conduct themselves in a manner that is worthy of esteem. "Respect" in Eastern culture is a bit more than the Western concept of politeness, that is, just being courteous. Good manners are rooted in sincerity and are practiced as a show of respect rather than an effort to avoid offending.

6. Integrity

A strong moral principle of holding to a high ethical standard. It is derived from qualities such as honesty, virtue, and consistency of character. A Samurai warrior was expected to make the right choices and do the right thing even if alone.

7. Duty (Loyalty)

A sense of commitment or obligation. True warriors are faithful and trustworthy.

8. Self-Control

Disciplined control of emotions and behavior in the face of impulses or temptations. True patience is many times considered bearing the unbearable. These warriors knew the difference between right and wrong as an absolute moral code and acted accordingly. There was little need for a police force in this feudal culture as self-control along with other aspects of the code were drivers of conduct and justice.

The Samurai didn't just consider Bushido a code. It wasn't something that was initially codified in written word. It was the warrior's way of life. Although there were intellectuals among the Samurai who thought deeply on these subjects, as intellect was highly valued, a Samurai was fundamentally a man of action.

This code was followed so strongly that in some ways adhering to it led to their destruction. It is paradoxical, but many Japanese officials did not adhere to this code of honor and helped push the Samurai class into historical legend. The Samurai would rather die than act in any way that didn't follow this code. So when faced with corrupt government, they accepted death instead of compromising their code. Principles mattered to the Samurai.

This seems irrational in Western culture. But a Samurai was honor bound to act even if the Samurai knew he would lose. Victory or defeat was not given a thought, only action, even if that action meant sacrifice.

LIFE AND DEATH

There is much philosophy surrounding death when studying the Samurai. Codes of honor were certainly matters of life and death to the Samurai. They were a warrior class of warlords and professional soldiers. They detached themselves from fear of death by accepting it as a part of life. Acting in accordance with their honorable code held more importance. Even the very word *Samurai* means "to serve." They put service over self-preservation and were indifferent to things like life and death. This concept starkly differentiates the Samurai from any other warrior culture.

Self-preservation is usually an instinct for a warrior. Separating themselves from concern over self-preservation is a defining trait of the Samurai, who took Bushido to a level few warriors can fathom.

Maybe it was the introduction of firearms that required less courage and skill in battle than the use of a sword that led to the change in how the code and culture changed for the Samurai. Maybe it was the absolute devotion the Samurai had toward the Bushido code without consideration for their own lives. The disappearance of the Samurai culture coincided with the abolishment of the feudal system after the fall of the Tokugawa shogunate and the Meiji Restoration of 1868. Whatever the ultimate reason, the Bushido code still exists but is practiced at a much different level than was exhibited by the Samurai of old.

Since much of the martial sense of honor originates from romanticized history of warriors such as the Samurai, Spartans, and Knights of the Round Table, who all adhered to similar codes of honor as warriors, the question always becomes, Were the Ninja warriors without honor?

It is a valid question, as Ninja were masters at winning fights. Determining if they were thugs or warriors is difficult, as their history is murky.

Ninja Honor

The Ninja, or Shinobi, were utilized as mercenaries and covert agents. They engaged in guerrilla warfare. Their unorthodox methods lead many to believe that these feudal warriors did not follow an honorable code of conduct. But they actually did have a code, and in reality, the Ninja complemented the Samurai.

The Bushido Code restricted the Samurai in certain circumstances. The reason was that Bushido wasn't just about fighting. Bushido was a way of life and arose from religious tenets as well. But in war there is this principle of winning at any cost, which may conflict with the Samurai's principles of daily conduct. The Samurai understood this quite well, as they were masters at winning fights but held to strict honorable methods. Sometimes they needed someone to do necessary work that was not very tidy.

The Ninja on the other hand were bound by a code to win at any cost, irrespective of the method required to win. The Samurai appreciated this aspect of the Ninja and sometimes hired them to perform dirty work on their behalf.[7]

This isn't to suggest the Ninja did not have a code of honor. Honor is often defined as behaving in a manner that is morally correct or doing what is right. The problem is that what is considered moral or correct may differ between cultures. This is the difference in honor as perceived by the Samurai and Ninja. There is no conflict in their sense of honor. It is simply that their perspectives were different.

What was not morally acceptable to the Samurai may have been morally acceptable to the Ninja, or any other culture for that matter. The concept of honor differs between cultures and may differ over time as well. Culture influences values.

The Samurai may have felt it was acceptable to kill an opponent because their lord had declared the opponent their enemy for nearly any reason. Simply because the lord wished the opponent killed, the Samurai was honor bound to execute the command. The Samurai were loyal soldiers. Samurai honor should still be considered honor, but the variables of ethical shifts must be considered when viewing it from afar.

Ninja were honor bound to protect their families or clans and had a strong sense of duty. But it is thought that most were not part of the formal social class system. Some could get work as Samurai and many Samurai worked as Ninja. Some Ninja may have been disgraced Samurai who had lost in battle or fled. But most were simply from villages and had a duty to protect their family and community. This is why most Ninja strongholds were in rural regions.

The distinctions were probably more fluid than history admits. But clearly Ninja were outsiders, and therefore their allegiance was to their clan and family. There was still a sense of honor, but from a different perspective. Honor and loyalty were focused on the clan rather than a lord. In this sense, Ninja were more independent in thought and action.

TRUE HONOR

Warriors throughout history have followed a code of honor. The concept of honor never changes. The way each warrior views what is honorable in accordance with their culture causes a difference in perception of honor.

To be clear on the subject, "honor killings" is a term in some ancient cultures that does not meet the definition of honor in other societies. It is misnamed. It should not use the word honor.

The homicide of someone due to a belief that shame has been brought on the family or there has been some violation of community principles does not necessarily meet the definition of honor in most cultures. It is simply homicide. Despite the term, it also has nothing to do with honor in the classic sense. The name is misleading to objective observers and is no small issue. The Honour Based Violence Awareness Network reports 5,000 honor killings a year perpetrated by family members, a practice denounced by the United Nations, which has stated that there is no honor in killing.[8] According to The Voice of the Martyrs, which tracks data over 67 nations, many individuals are imprisoned or persecuted simply for their beliefs.[9]

This is why the modern definition of honor struggles to capture the true sense of the concept. Honor clearly is being true to a set of values that represents integrity. True honor is a deep concept that cannot be sullied by individual perceptions or cultures, which may have a twisted view of honor.

The depth of honor may also have been watered down through generations. Historically, many have been willing to die for honor.

True honor is something America's founding fathers died for, as have others who fought for freedom throughout history. Honor is more meaningful than superficial definitions or cultural perceptions. It is beyond oneself and it rises above changing societal norms.

There are many who wish to be right. But there are few who admit when they are wrong. True honor is having the courage to do what is right and to admit when you are wrong. True honor is reflective of how the warrior treats others, corrects his wrongs, and strives to do the right thing in all situations. This is honor that can be humbling.

CLASSICAL HONOR

Honor in the classical sense is a reputation that is worthy of admiration and respect as judged by others. Members of a group set minimum standards for behavior. Those meeting the standards earn the mutual respect of the group. Rising above these standards earns more respect. But members of the group hold each other accountable in this classical sense. A football team or combat unit is made stronger by a sense of honor and commitment among its members. But honor is largely being lost in a more global anonymous society. Fraternal organizations, fire departments, and police departments are some of the last groups along with teams and the military that understand a sense of this classical definition of honor.

Anthropologist Julian Pitt-Rivers has written that honor isn't simply each person's perception of their own value; it is the perception of others as well.[10] Before modern laws this sense of honor governed behavior. Honor was motivational and protected society. So guarding one's reputation was important as a driver of behavior.

The decline in face-to-face relationships in modern times has decreased the value of honor. A culture of honor has less worth with urbanization, impersonal interactions, and anonymity on the rise. Individual unethical or immoral behavior is less likely to be noticed. People are less likely to put aside their personal needs or values for the common good in a more diverse society, as an increasingly global civilization blurs the meaning of common good. The culture of modern society is more one of "to each his own." Boundaries are not defined as much by national borders as by regions of thought.

In a modern society it also is less feasible to defend one's honor with violence. Boys can no longer settle disputes on the playground then continue being friends afterward. Adults must intervene. You cannot punch someone or challenge someone to a duel in defense of honor. Any intertwining of honor with violence in a litigious society is no longer acceptable. Disputes cannot be settled physically.

As a result, honor has received bad press in modern times outside pockets of organizations where honor is still valued. Traditional honor was believed to incite violence in the past, creating intolerance to a more open society according to this evolving new world view. The idea that honor is what drove good behavior in society for centuries is lost with this new thinking.

Honor carries a code of moral conduct with it in a time when morality is also suffering from a blurring of definition. Honor is when someone acts not out of obedience or because someone is looking but from a personal code of conduct. It is doing something not simply because it is the law, but because it is right. There was a time when honor was more important than law in shaping behavior and society. So while there certainly is secular morality, there was once less of a debate about what was good and what was moral without a foundational structure. There simply seems to be less internal guidance in regard to what constitutes ethical behavior in modern times. Honor was once the glue that held many civilizations together.

Honor combats incompetence and corruption. If rules and law were the only guides for behavior then individuals would do the least they could and still avoid violating the rules or law. This creates mediocrity. Society has become more complex, and the principles of honor are more important than ever to govern behavior.

A warrior living by a code of honor should not be a rarity in modern society. Having a code of honor means the warrior's sense of ethics isn't situational. Honor is living with integrity and a sense of justice that transcends modern superficial views of what is right. These values are nonnegotiable to the warrior.

Honor is therefore necessary to prevent a warrior from becoming corrupted by modern society and its values and ethics, which waver with time. Medieval knights had a code of chivalry. The warrior code of Bushido governed the conduct of the Samurai. The ancient Spartans possessed similar codes of behavior. The French Foreign Legion of today follows the *code d'honeur*. Honor is what defines the warrior and sets him apart from the rest of society.

Retired marine General James Mattis testified before Congress on January 12, 2017. He echoed a belief that America has two fundamental powers. One is the power of intimidation. The other power is inspiration. As a marine, he was part of the intimidation side of the power equation for most of his career. His belief was that inspiration should be employed more often.

While many principles of fighting certainly emerge from the power of intimidation, honor has the power of inspiration. It is another power the warrior has at his or her disposal to influence the world.

Honor is something our fathers taught us. It is something we should teach our children. It is a quality fighters must possess to be great.

Notes

1. Travis Smith, "Proverbs 21:10–11—'There is no honor among thieves,'" *Travis Smith Blog*, June 21, 2014, https://heartofashepherd.com/2014/06/21/proverbs-2110-11-there-is-no-honor-among-thieves/.
2. Ed Grabianowski, "How Samurai Work," *HowStuffWorks.com*, April 16, 2004, http://people.howstuffworks.com/samurai5.htm.
3. Inazo Nitobe, *Bushido: The Code of the Samurai* (Birmingham, AL: Cliff Road Books, 2006).
4. Miles Menander Dawson, *The Ethics of Confucius* (Honolulu, HI: The University Press of the Pacific, 1915), http://www.sacred-texts.com/cfu/eoc/eoc06.htm.
5. "Hector: Greek Mythology," *Encyclopædia Britannica* (2014), https://www.britannica.com/topic/Hector-Greek-mythology.
6. Francois de La Rochefocauld, "Quotationspage," *Michael Moncur's Quotations*, n.d., http://www.quotationspage.com/quote/32971.html.
7. "Martial Art," *Encyclopædia Britannica* (2017), https://www.britannica.com/sports/martial-art#ref36127; Kallie Szczepanski, "The Ninja of Japan," *Thoughtco.com* (2017), https://www.thoughtco.com/history-of-the-ninja-195811.

8. Honour Based Violence Awareness Network, *International Resource Centre*, n.d., http://hbv-awareness.com.

9. The Voice of the Martyrs, *About the Voice of the Martyrs*, https://www.persecution.com.

10. Julian Pitt-Rivers, "Honor," in *International Encyclopedia of the Social Sciences* 18 vols., ed. David L. Sills (New York: Macmillan, 1968), 503–511.

武器

FIGHTING WITH WEAPONS

WEAPONS ARE AN extension of the fighter. The Samurai even considered the sword to be an extension of their souls. The weapon assumes the character of whoever wields it, as the weapon is simply a tool that extends the will of the fighter. The principles of fighting with empty hands also apply to fighting with weapons. A fight is a fight. But there are some thoughts about these principles that should be noted.

A weapon is a great equalizer and a force multiplier. A sufficiently armed weak or elderly person can repel the attack of a much stronger attacker or multiple aggressors. A weapon can save lives and prevent injury if an attack is prevented by this show of force.

Revealing that the victim has a weapon can discourage an attacker from causing injury in many cases. Even a fighter capable of effective unarmed combat who possesses a weapon might be able to avoid a fight if the attacker believes the fighter has a weapon that multiplies the fighter's effectiveness. An aggressor may be willing to take his chances with a fighter in an unarmed engagement. But if the aggressor thinks a weapon may become engaged he may change his mind and seek an easier target. The balance of power shifts the odds dramatically when weapons are employed.

Weapons make up for size. Police officers must sometimes fill out a use of force form every time they use physical force to restrain an offender. One particular officer at a local police department where I used to work was a small guy. He was called into the chief's office one day because he had more use of force forms on file than the rest of the department combined.

The small officer told the chief to take a look at how big he was compared to the other officers. When the large officers went to arrest someone, offenders complied easily. But when he tried to arrest someone, offenders thought they could overpower the officer because the officer would be judicious with his use of weapons. Therefore, he got into more fights because he is smaller. A criminal will target victims he perceives as easy prey who can be overpowered. A weapon changes that balance of power.

Criminals in prison have been interviewed in order to learn what deters them most from committing crimes. Consistently, criminals cite armed victims as the greatest deterrent.

The Centers for Disease Control came to a similar conclusion in 2013 as part of a $10 million study commissioned by President Obama. According to their research, "Studies that directly assessed the effect of actual defensive uses of guns (i.e., incidents in which a gun was 'used' by the crime victim in the sense of attacking or threatening an offender) have found consistently lower injury rates among gun-using crime victims compared with victims who used other self-protective strategies." The study goes on to say that almost all national estimates reveal defensive use of guns by victims is as common as offensive uses by criminals.[1]

Carrying and deploying a weapon should be a thoughtful process. One should never carry a weapon without being trained in its use. A weapon should also not be carried if you are not willing to use it if necessary. Otherwise, you've just brought a weapon for the aggressor to use against you.

A knife is the most common carry weapon. Laws should be examined in the area the knife will be carried in order to ensure compliance with local laws.

In a fight, a knife should be felt, not seen. It is why a rapid deployment system must be considered. In other words, a knife that deploys as it is pulled from the pocket. Openly wielding a knife surrenders the element of surprise in counterattack. It should be deployed or held at the ready in a manner that preserves this element. In other words, the knife should be held in a hidden posture if possible as waving it around only works in the movies. It can't be said enough that a knife should be felt, not seen. There also is a high probability that both fighters will be cut in a fight between two knife-wielding fighters regardless of who wins.

Likewise, a gun should not be deployed unless it is necessary to shoot someone. Pulling it out has certainly resulted in deterrence and prevented many altercations. But it should not come out only for display. It should be deployed only if there is sufficient cause to fire the weapon and the person carrying the weapon must be willing to use it or the weapon should never be deployed. Training to use a handgun is probably the path of least resistance when deciding how best to protect yourself.

Do not extend a gun toward an assailant if he is close. You are just offering the weapon to him. Maintain enough distance to protect the weapon. Competing in the Self-Defense Division of Martial Arts Tournaments for many years, it was fun practicing weapon disarms. You'd be surprised how quickly a trained fighter can take a weapon away from someone. Don't think inmates in prison don't practice these same techniques. Seek training on carrying, using, and firing the weapon. This training should include weapon retention as well. You must also know area laws regarding what weapons can be carried and license requirements for concealment if applicable.

Although a knife and gun are the most common weapons that come to mind, weapons are essentially limitless. Anything that aids in gaining a strategic, physical, or mental advantage over an opponent is a weapon.

Ordinary objects can become weapons. Pencils, lamps, marbles, cars, and fierce words have all been used as diverse weapons. Weapons then escalate in scale to biological, cyber, and ballistic missiles. For example, a stick is an effective and innocuous weapon.

Known as escrima, kali, or arnis, stick fighting is the national martial art of the Philippines.[2] This weapon-based system uses sticks and bladed weapons. Many students in the Filipino Martial Arts system learn to fight with weapons first before advancing to empty-handed combat. The muscle memory in both is essentially the same. It also conditions practitioners to fight against armed opponents.

A pair of sticks is usually utilized, which forces the fighter to be ambidextrous. These sticks extend the reach and power of the fighter and are always moving in different directions. The constant motion increases velocity, confuses the opponent, and minimizes telegraphing where you will strike.

Range and striking force are significantly increased using escrima sticks. If given a choice, many trained practitioners would choose a stick over a knife in many circumstances. A knife is certainly deadly. But a knife requires a closer range to be effective. The longer range of the stick can hold a knife-wielding attacker at bay if used properly. Therefore, not only the lethality of the weapon should be considered, but the range at which it is lethal must be considered as well.

One of the deadliest bladed weapons used by fighters of the Filipino arts is the karambit. It is a small knife from Southeast Asia that is curved and intended to mimic an animal's claw. The destructive force it delivers in such a small package serves as a reminder as to why claws are slightly curved in nature.

Another feature of the karambit is a ring guard opposite the blade end. A finger is inserted, which makes it difficult to disarm someone using a karambit. It was originally a farming implement and became more curved as it was weaponized. It is the perfect weapon for a police officer to carry on his weak side to help protect the weapon on his strong side. It can be deployed quickly in a single motion, but those carrying a karambit must first understand its proper deployment and use. Doug Marcaida, a judge on the History Channel's *Forged in Fire*, is an expert in these stick and edged-weapon arts.[3] He is a credible source on the use of these weapons.

Peasants in Southeast Asia and other parts of the world were the first to use these types of implements as weapons. Farming tools were the closest items at hand. While the Samurai were warriors who carried and trained with swords each day, farmers used anything at their disposal. We could list many martial arts weapons that started in this manner. For example, the nunchaku was a threshing tool used by Okinawan farmers. Bruce Lee popularized its use as a weapon.

Today a pencil at a desk is a weapon. A key chain is a weapon. As in the earliest cultures, everyday items can be utilized for protection.

RIGHTS

The right to self-protection should be self-evident. The U.S. Constitution guarantees the individual the right to bear arms with the specific purpose of protecting citizens against tyranny. Unfortunately, this tyranny can come from governments, as evidenced through history. The right to self-defense has existed since the dawn of civilization.

Most cultures and societies over time recognized the right to bear weapons or act in self-preservation. In early Rome, Cicero argued that the right to self-defense was inborn and not a creation of government.[4] John Locke argued in 1690 that civil government properly exists to protect individuals.[5] Thomas Jefferson agreed and the Constitution was designed to not only protect citizens but to also protect citizens from government, which has been a problem throughout history as regimes become powerful and evil. In fact, disarming citizens is one of the first acts necessary to overcome a population.

The U.S. Supreme Court, in *United States v. Verdugo-Urquidez*,[6] indicated that the word "people" in the Second Amendment referred to individuals, not states. The language of the Constitution prohibits the federal government from infringing on those rights and is as clear on this point as in the prohibition of infringing on the First Amendment rights to free speech, press, and religious expression.

According to the Court, a comma is what protects the right to bear arms for individuals. The Second Amendment reads, "A well regulated Militia, being necessary to the security of a free State, the right of the people to keep and bear arms, shall not be infringed." That comma after "the security of a free State," divides the amendment into two clauses according to the D.C. Circuit Court of Appeals and the Supreme Court, both of which struck down the District of Columbia's gun ban. The first part is "prefatory" or throat clearing as noted by some, as security of a free state is necessary.

But then the Constitution writers get down to business with the "operative" clause that the right of the people to bear arms shall not be infringed.

The little comma has the power of "and" as no other word makes sense. The Constitution was drafted with great care. A well-regulated militia "and" the right of the people to keep and bear arms is the only meaning that makes sense with the comma. Using other words (of, or) is nonsensical as the writing style of the day usually provided a preamble before certain main thoughts. Under examination, the right to bear arms isn't limited to just militias, and now the courts agree.[7]

This point must be clear. Groups wishing to ban guns say the comma is just a pause to catch your breath while reading the amendment and that only militias should have guns. The courts disagree with this view.

The amendment is divided not to indicate a pause in its reading, but to contrast the militia and the people. A well-regulated militia is necessary. But the right of the people in contrast should not be infringed. It doesn't say the rights of the militia shall not be infringed. It says the right of the people should not be infringed.

The people who wrote the Constitution had just fought a war against armed militias from a tyrannical state. The writers knew they might have to fight again one day. So they made the possession of weapons a right that the militia could not take away.

Much of the work in designing our system of government revolved around protecting the people from the government. We have different branches of government to balance power and many mechanisms in place to prevent a recurrence of what the framers of the Constitution had just gone through. So let's be clear that the Second Amendment is about citizens protecting themselves against a future tyrannical government. That was fresh on the framers' minds as they wrote those protections into the Constitution. They knew that disarming the populace was the first step a tyrannical government would take to control citizens. It has happened throughout history. But the framers of the Constitution wanted to make sure it didn't happen here.

REALITY

Aggressors understand the power of weapons. While we debate the right of being armed for protection or to guard against tyranny, evil men disregard this debate. They will be armed regardless of what the law establishes as legal boundaries in regard to arms. Gun-free zones are where most shootings occur. These zones make it easy for criminals who disregard laws. Cities with the most gun control laws typically have some of the highest gun crime rates. Again, criminals disregard laws.

Most homicides involve weapons.[8] Around half of all robberies involve weapons. Nearly a quarter of assaults involve weapons. Weapons increase the likelihood of injury and come into play often in confrontations.

Understand that criminals do not want a fight. They consider a fight as something that has rules or is engaged between two equally skilled opponents. If criminals are looking for a fight, they want a fight they know they can win. Criminals want an easy victim. They wish to ambush and win without a fight or at least an easy fight. This is why gun-free zones are a welcome sight to criminals. This is why criminals target easy prey.

This gives credence to the view that there are two types of people in the world: predators and prey. A predator isn't going to bother another predator. He might get hurt. A predator seeks prey. A predator wants to stack the deck in his favor.

Criminals do not wish to use weapons to fight per se. They use weapons to tilt power in their favor and win easily. The last thing a criminal wants is a fight on equal terms. If an attacker wanted a fight he wouldn't have attacked you with a weapon. He just wants to overwhelm you in order to commit a crime more easily. A weapon gives a criminal this power.

We've heard the movie line that if he pulls out a knife, you pull out a gun. There is little fight in this escalation of arms. The idea is to have the superior weapon to win, not fight. Criminals know this. They want the superior weapon at their disposal at the time.

So while you consider fighting with weapons, it also must be considered that your opponent may be armed as well. An armed conflict must always be considered and heightens the importance of the principles of winning fights, specifically the principles of preparation and awareness.

Krav maga founder Imi Sde-Or and many other analysts have observed that victims of violent attacks against knife-wielding aggressors consistently reported that they were unaware that a weapon was involved in the fight until after they had received laceration wounds.[9] The victims thought they were involved in an unarmed fight. It wasn't until after they sustained significant injury that they realized their opponent was armed. Knife fights are fast, quick, and lethal.

This is the true essence of fighting with weapons. Again, a weapon like a knife should typically be felt, not seen, and that's precisely what happens. Weapons tilt the balance of power so heavily that the fight may be over before you know it has begun. This is why you never let anyone get too close—especially if they may have a weapon, and any weapon will fall into this category. Always control the space around you and your distance from potential threats.

TUELLER RULE

How close is dangerous? The answer to that question is always the Tueller rule.

Sergeant Dennis Tueller was a police officer with the Salt Lake City Police Department. A drill named after Tueller was first described in his 1983 article in *S.W.A.T.* magazine, "How Close Is Too Close?"[10]

Tueller had conducted tests that demonstrated people of various heights, weights, and ages could close the distance of 21 feet in an average of 1.5 seconds. That's about the length of time it takes a highly trained officer to draw his handgun and fire an aimed shot.

Keep in mind that someone who is shot doesn't fall instantly like in the movies. They can still be a threat for a few moments or few feet after being shot. Tueller concluded that a person armed with a knife or other handheld weapon was a potential lethal threat, even at 21 feet away. That's right, even a knife against a firearm.

If a knife-wielding attacker is 21 feet away the victim with a firearm must draw, shoot, and quickly move away to avoid injury. Footwork and movement are still important even if defending with a firearm. A knife-wielding attacker is still dangerous to someone carrying a gun at that distance. There is an old saying among shooters that if you're not shooting you must be moving.

So always assume someone else has a weapon and do not let him or her get too close. Anything less than 21 feet away is too close. Keep moving and don't let the attacker close the distance even if they have a knife and you have a gun.

APPLICATION

Tactical application of weaponry mirrors that of unarmed principles. You must still decide which weapons you will carry to protect yourself and your family, then prepare to use these weapons through training.

Awareness is still key, and as the Tueller rule illustrates, this awareness must encompass not allowing any threat to get close. The very first tactical application of armed or unarmed self-defense is maintaining distance, which involves being aware of surroundings and potential threats.

Commitment to the proper deployment of the weapon is also key. You must be committed or willing to use the weapon and be willing to exercise the maximum lethal potential of that weapon.

The remainder of the principles must fall into place as well. Efficiency with the weapon, discipline, power, focus, and ferocity will help win a fight with a weapon. Simply having a weapon will many times accomplish the principle of surprise, as an attacker probably would not have attacked knowing that you possessed a weapon.

It can't be said enough that a weapon is a force multiplier. Even throwing debris or anything nearby at hand can be used as a weapon. But the principles of winning a fight are the same in an armed fight as they are in an unarmed fight.

COMBAT MIND-SET

Lt. Col. Jeff Cooper's 1988 book, *To Ride, Shoot Straight, and Speak the Truth*,[11] summed up what he referred to as the combat mind-set to win a fight.

Cooper was an expert on gun fighting. But the principles he applied in his gun-fighting classes apply to both armed and unarmed combat. He believed that gunfights were not won by dexterity, skill, or even marksmanship. They were won by what he called a combat mind-set, which he said was composed of awareness, anticipation, concentration, and coolness. Cooper summed up centuries of fight principles in those four words.

The combat mind-set is simply being aware that if a weapon must be deployed to help win a fight that the reaction is not one of shock but of control. This is a reasonable view that only comes through advanced preparation and training.

A fighter shouldn't be surprised by finding that a situation is out of control. A fighter should develop a mind-set that he is in control and the situation is not controlled by the aggressor or opponent.

Cooper specifically believed that if someone was trying to kill you that the combat mind-set would not result in a feeling of fear but a feeling of wrathful anger. This is why the principle of ferocity may best be represented as primal rage against a threat. Steadied by the other principles, this rage is concentrated, disciplined, and efficient.

The combat mind-set helps condition a fighter to respond in what can only be described as a professional manner to end the conflict. When someone is shooting at you, the professional response is to focus on your own shooting. This is the coolness Lt. Col. Cooper was trying to get across. Focus on the front sight of the weapon during the situation at hand and nothing more.

In Cooper's research, police officers that focused on their front sight hit their targets. Those who never paid attention to their front sight and lost focus missed. It all involves mind-set. It also must be noted that Cooper advocated four basic gun safety rules that now have become universal and should be mentioned when having a discussion about firearms:

1. All guns should be considered loaded even if they are not loaded.
2. Never let the muzzle point toward anything you are not willing to destroy.
3. Keep the finger off the trigger until the sights are on the target and you are ready to fire.
4. Identify not only the target before firing, but also what is behind it. Know what you are going to shoot before you fire.

Six-time International Practical Shooting Confederation World Champion Rob Leatham[12] would add that not moving the gun is another secret to accurate shooting. If you move the gun, aiming is useless. Leatham has advised that if you shoot fast you're going to jerk the trigger. Just learn to jerk the trigger without moving the gun. He says it's simple, but it's not easy to do. Aiming only matters when you don't move the gun.

Leatham's advice is simply:

1. Hold the gun tight.
2. Point the gun at the target.
3. Pull the trigger without moving the gun.

WINNING WITH WEAPONS

The way to win a fight is to realize there may be a fight before it occurs. With this concept, you get to pick your weapon and dictate some of the rules of the conflict ahead of time.

You need to know that the world is a dangerous place and what to expect. This will help guide your selection of weapon and training to meet that challenge. You also need to understand your level of skill with weapons. Do not carry something you cannot effectively deploy.

You must always be careful. This isn't fear, it's caution. If you don't realize that you are vulnerable or in trouble then no amount of skill will make up for that lack of knowledge and preparation. That is why preparation and awareness are the first principles. Weapons can end a conflict very quickly and be over before you know it. But this works both ways. It can end quickly for the assailant or the victim. Do not be careless when you are armed or when your assailant is possibly armed.

Finally, the proper weapon to carry is the one you will carry. It sounds simple, but understand that you can possess an awesome knife or firearm but if you don't have it with you when a fight occurs then it is useless.

NOTES

1. Alissa Tabirian, "CDC Study: Use of Firearms for Self-Defense is 'Important Crime Deterrent,'" *CNSNews.com*, July 17, 2013, http://www.cnsnews.com /news/article/cdc-study-use-firearms-self-defense-important-crime-deterrent; Alan I. Leshner et al., *Priorities for Research to Reduce the Threat of Firearm-Related Violence* (Washington, DC: The National Academies Press, 2013).
2. Robert Young, "FMA 101: A Practical Primer on the Filipino Martial Arts," *Black Belt Magazine*, April 4, 2017, http://www.blackbeltmag.com/category /escrima/.
3. History Channel, "Doug Marcaida Bios," *A&E Network* (2017), http://www .history.com/shows/forged-in-fire/cast/doug-marcaida.

4. Jan Hessbruegge, *Human Rights and Personal Self-Defense in International Law* (Oxford, UK: Oxford University Press, 2017), 30–31.

5. Alex Tuckness, "Locke's Political Philosophy," *The Stanford Encyclopedia of Philosophy* (2016), https://plato.stanford.edu/entries/locke-political/.

6. United States v. Verdugo-Urquidez, 494 U.S. 259 (U.S. Court of Appeals for the Ninth Circuit 1990), https://www.oyez.org/cases/1989/88-1353.

7. Adam Freedman, "Clause and Effect," *New York Times*, December 16, 2007.

8. Alexia Cooper and Erica Smith, *Homicide Trends in the US, 1980–2008* (Washington, DC: U.S. Department of Justice, 2011).

9. Patrice Bonnafoux, "Self-Defence against Knife Attacks: A Full Review," *Urbanfitandfearless Blog*, n.d., http://www.urbanfitandfearless.com/2016/09/self-defence-against-knife-attacks.html.

10. Ron Marinelli, "Revisiting the 21 Foot Rule," *Policemag.com*, September 18, 2014, http://www.policemag.com/channel/weapons/articles/2014/09/revisiting-the-21-foot-rule.aspx; Dennis Tueller, "How Close Is Too Close?" *S.W.A.T. Magazine*, March 1983.

11. Jeff Cooper, *To Ride, Shoot Straight, and Speak the Truth* (Boulder, CO: Paladin Press, 1988).

12. Rob Leatham, n.d., http://robleatham.com.

言葉

リーダー武蔵

FIGHTING WITH
WORDS

A MONK ASKED the chief priest if he could smoke while he prayed. The chief priest denied the request. Another monk asked the chief priest if he could pray while he smoked. The chief priest agreed to the request from the second monk.[1]

The ultimate result was that both monks were doing the exact same thing. They both had the intention of smoking and praying at the same time. But each framed their words to the chief priest differently and received different responses. This is the power of words and framing those words. The power of words is understood and utilized by many methods such as cognitive bias, misdirection, or framing. Warriors may not like the fact that words are also weapons, but the concept isn't new. In fact, words are typically the first weapons drawn during a fight.

As mentioned earlier, a Samurai warrior possessed a mushin mind-set. Again, though *mushin* is sometimes translated as "disinterested," it doesn't mean uninterested. It means the Samurai approached activity in a dispassionate manner or with an unbiased mind-set. He wasn't easily moved by words. He was flexible and had a calm, still center. This concept is especially applicable to fighting with words.

When under verbal assault, a fighter must be like a willow tree, which bends and survives heavy winds by its flexibility. It is the same approach taught by aikido, jujutsu, and judo. Using an opponent's strength against him has power. Controlling a situation by acting in a malleable manner is adapting to different levels of cognitive bias, intelligence, or behavior. Like aikido, deflection and redirection work much better than direct confrontation, even in verbal assaults.

Verbal attack expects disagreement. When a verbal attack is confronted with agreement in some fashion, the verbal attacker doesn't know what to do, as the response is disarming.

Finding any semblance of common ground, accepting what comes and dealing with it calmly and dispassionately requires quite a bit of discipline. This discipline can be in short supply during modern times but it comes from contentment with oneself. We find this wisdom in many ancient philosophies from Buddhism, to Taoism and Christianity.

Worrying or getting upset in a verbal confrontation doesn't change a hair on anyone's head. Submission to life's hardships in the sense that hardships, harsh words, and challenges are a natural part of life disarms words of much of their power over you.

This doesn't mean to take words or challenges lying down. It simply means it is better to ride out a wave in a storm than fight against the water and drown. It was this notion that Yamamoto Tsunetomo had in mind where his thoughts were written in *The Hagakure*: "There is something about a rainstorm. When meeting with a sudden shower, you try not to get wet and run quickly along the road. But doing such things as passing under eaves of houses, you still get wet. When you are resolved from the beginning, you will not be perplexed, though you still get the same soaking. This understanding extends to everything."[2]

Moshe ben Maimon was a twelfth-century Jewish rabbi famous for saying one should accept the truth from whatever source it proceeds.[3] There are numerous sources throughout ancient literature that urge calmness of spirit and mind in the face of conflict. Truth is truth.

When it rains, accept that you will get wet. Accept that words are often meant to be painful. Accepting certain truths eases internal tension. Calmness provides you with an edge when words are drawn as weapons.

IN THE DOJO

I was still in high school when I started martial arts training. Master Thompson was my sensei and a PKA State Champion Full Contact Kickboxer. Naturally, we sparred during most classes, as that was his specialty. He was an intimidating fighter with long arms and well-defined muscles. I was far from intimidating.

I wore glasses. So I had to take them off to spar and got pretty good at sparing after a while. I'd take a punch even if I halfway blocked it and would keep fighting. I tried to be tough as I was one of the smaller guys in the class. Without glasses I couldn't see some of the action that was just a blur. My strategy was to simply stand my ground, withstand the blows, and keep fighting against those who clearly were more intimidating.

Then I heard about contact lenses and that fighters could wear them while fighting. This sounded great, so I was fitted for contact lenses. I was excited to try them out during class, as sparring was just a blur of visual activity for me without glasses.

Master Thompson lined us up. Wearing contacts my vision was clear. He gave the command "*Hajime,*" which is the Japanese term he used to begin. My sparring partner whom I had stood toe to toe fighting in the past lunged toward me with a punch. Only this time, I didn't stand toe to toe. I backed up—a lot.

"*Yame,*" Master Thompson commanded us to stop the fight. I hadn't backed up before and he wondered if everything was okay. It occurred to me that my sparring partner was trying to hit me. I saw the punch coming clearly with my new contacts in place. There was no longer a blur.

When I could only see a blur, I wasn't afraid of the punch. It was just a blur. I'd block or let it graze me and keep going. Now that I could see clearly, the thought of getting hit was worse than being hit. I had never really seen a punch coming at me full speed before. That was the first time and I was a bit amazed at the clarity.

As a young martial artist, I quickly overcame this temporary setback. And I guess it was best to start out not being able to see well in order to learn a punch doesn't hurt as bad as you'd think. But the lesson was as clear as the vision of punches. The thought of being hit is worse than actually being hit. Words are the same way.

PAINFUL WORDS

A good fighter accepts he will be hit during a fight. Therefore, an opponent's punch that breaks through his defenses doesn't startle the fighter as he has already accepted getting hit is part of fighting. Accepting the reality that harmful words are used as weapons today is no different. Dealing with words may need to be dealt with in a more artful manner, however, such as how aikido deals with a punch. But in the end, the thought of the word is what hurts, not the word. The word only hurts if you allow it to hurt.

A powerful martial artist may be able to overpower an opponent physically through sheer skill. But words used as weapons generally come in unlimited supply and are untiring. Verbal conflict is more about defusing and redirecting. It is more like aikido or judo than a hard style that meets the confrontation head on.

Now there is verbal war as well. Never confuse the two. Verbal conflict is when words are simply the preamble to violence. This needs to be de-escalated before it becomes physical. There are techniques to attempt this de-escalation.

However, verbal war is the word fight. The person may not necessarily desire it to be physical. The words are not meant for escalation or testing the boundaries of the other person. The words are the primary weapons and are meant to destroy. Verbal war is less likely to be de-escalated, as the aggressor wants a verbal fight and nothing more.

Actually, when in doubt, verbal defense in a calm manner is the best approach as guided by ancient wisdom in dealing with either situation. There are many ways to accomplish it.

FEEL, FELT, FOUND

I know how you feel. I've felt the same way. But here's what I've found. It is one of many deflection techniques to redirect verbal attacks and win or defuse a verbal confrontation. Acknowledging the other person's view is of primary importance in this redirection. Then admit you understand their view. And finally introduce another option.

Most people simply want to be heard. They want to be asked rather than told and they want to know why they are being asked to do something rather than receive demands. They want options, not threats.

Listen, Empathize, Ask, Paraphrase, and Summarize (LEAPS) is another technique to deflect verbal escalation noted by George Thompson and Jerry Jenkins in their book, *Verbal Judo*.[4] Listening to an angry person takes patience. But it also allows them to expend emotional energy. A fighter simply enters a state of mushin, finding a calm center to listen dispassionately. He listens, but the words are simply information and do not inflame the warrior to the degree they do for someone who lacks the mushin mind-set. It is a concept found in many of the world's religions. Turning the other cheek. Responding to harsh words with soft words. These responses require self-discipline and take the sting out of words.

Everyone wants to be treated with dignity and respect. Expressing empathy helps. Ask for information respectfully, then paraphrase and summarize their thoughts to let them know you are listening. It is simply a way to work through a verbal confrontation.

WINNING

Sun Tzu is famous for saying that to win one hundred victories in one hundred battles is not the highest skill. To subdue an enemy without fighting is the highest skill. This places fighting with words as a primary tool in winning fights.

Most fights start with a verbal confrontation. Wars have started over words. Unless a criminal is simply hunting an easy target, a fight will typically start with words. Again, words are the first weapon of choice.

Another ancient Samurai saying is that when a man throws a spear of insult at your head, move your head. The spear will then miss its target leaving the attacker empty-handed. The spear is then in the wall, not in you.[5] (Sort of beats "sticks and stones will break your bones but words will never hurt you.") Ignoring or deflecting an insult disarms the power of the words, as they don't have their intended effect.

Swiss psychoanalyst Carl Jung (1875–1961) believed there are four stages of life: the athlete, the warrior, the statement (sometimes written as the statesman) and the spirit.[6] It's something to think about. Learning to deflect and de-escalate violence is a higher skill. The earliest years of life are represented by the athlete, who tends to be self-absorbed. Younger fighters simply want to fight. The warrior stage is when we begin to take on responsibilities and feel we want to conquer the world.

It isn't until later in life when we reach the statement stage when we ask ourselves what we have done for others. We've become parents and we wish to leave a legacy. We then pass into the spiritual stage, when we understand we are more than our possessions.

More experienced fighters have nothing to prove and have reached the statement or the spiritual level. Higher-level warriors have learned to avoid violence, as they are not self-absorbed or wishing to conquer the world. They understand situations at a higher level and do not bend to the lower levels of thinking.

DE-ESCALATION

Michael Kuhr was Germany's first world champion in kickboxing. He now runs a successful security company in Berlin known for its professionalism.[7] Some refer to Kuhr as *Der Pate*, which translates to "the godfather." His security business requires integrity, discipline, and a cool head when situations become tense. As a pro kickboxer, Kuhr certainly knows how to fight. There are few things he fears.

A video of Kuhr went viral with nearly 26 million views of the original, demonstrating his de-escalation skills and professionalism under fire. In the viral video, a loud patron trying to get into a club is denied access by one of Kuhr's security men. Kuhr is dressed in a suit and tie. He pulls the angry patron to the side politely saying he wants to speak with the man.

The entire time the man is shouting insults and profanities. Kuhr is unfazed as he gets the patron away from the crowd. The loudmouth screams at Kuhr saying he will screw him and his mother. The man is much taller than Kuhr and leans over Kuhr trying to intimidate the world kickboxing champion. Kuhr competed in the under-60-kilogram division and isn't very large. But he is known as one of the toughest full-contact kickboxers in the world. Kuhr is not someone a hothead should annoy.

Kuhr replies calmly that the man cannot do those things because his mother is too old for him. The calm response confuses the angry man. Kuhr adds that he is heterosexual so he can't screw him either adding that the man looks familiar. He thinks he knows the loudmouth. Kuhr is constantly and calmly redirecting the man.

The angry patron is clearly puzzled with Kuhr's calm matter-of-fact and even humorous responses. Screaming at Kuhr even more, he asks who does he think he is and how should he know him. Kuhr says he trained the loudmouth's brother and if the loudmouth doesn't behave Kuhr says he will call his brother and calls his brother's name.

The angry patron asks who Kuhr is again. Kuhr simply says Michael Kuhr. The angry patron then immediately recognizes who he is annoying. He calms down, realizing he is yelling at one of the toughest fighters in the world. Kuhr says he will accept an apology and not call his brother. The patron is very calm at this point and thanks Kuhr for not calling his brother. Kuhr shakes the man's hand and gives him some advice to behave or he won't get into any club. He allows the man an honorable way out of further confrontation.

The point is, Kuhr calmed the situation masterfully. Kuhr could have quickly beaten the man physically. The fight would have been quick and easy for someone with Kuhr's experience. But he didn't.

Kuhr could have gotten into a shouting match with the patron hurling his own obscenities. He could have ordered the man to calm down or provided other verbal assaults back at the man. But he didn't do this either.

Instead, Kuhr maintained his composure. He approached the man with the detached calm demeanor Samurai call mushin. He simply deflected the man's insults without being offended or offending the man in return. In fact, his responses were hilarious as well as unexpected.

Most importantly, Kuhr controlled the situation. He found a way to calm the man. He showed the angry patron respect and acted as if he was simply trying to help the man. If the man didn't behave he wouldn't get into any clubs and his brother would be disappointed in the way he was acting.[8]

In martial arts, we teach how to deflect punches. You can either block the punch or dodge out of the way. Either way is an effective way to avoid getting hit.

Calm answers to insults are a figurative way of blocking or dodging so as not to be affected by the insult. There is biblical instruction in

Proverbs 15:1 that a soft answer turns away wrath, but harsh words stir anger. A soft answer is simply a gentle answer. If you reply with anger then you are in the middle of an argument with the other angry person. An angry person cannot argue alone.

A pleasing tone is certainly difficult when someone is verbally hurling angry wrath your way. But a fighter must maintain composure. Theodore Roosevelt once said to speak softly but carry a big stick. Verbal violence is often a prelude to physical violence. So while one speaks softly, the fighter must be prepared for violence at any moment. De-escalating the fight at the verbal stage takes much less physical effort but a bit more mental effort.

Soft responses such as, "I understand, sir" or "Yes sir, I hear you" are simply ways to deflect the insult and focus on controlling the situation. These responses can then be the door to empower the person to help you de-escalate the anger. Following up the deflection with what you need them to do helps. Tell the person you will see what you can do to help or ask him or her to help you out by explaining the problem to a manager. Or even agree to disagree; whatever you need them to do in order to get a calm resolution or at least civil behavior rather than irrational action.

Keep in mind that some people are simply unreasonable. At the end of the day, as long as their words aren't inflaming their own anger even more, simply watch their behavior as much as their language. Telling them to calm down may incite them more if their words are fueling their own rage.

If the person is making threats, increasing his tone, or exhibiting other behavior signaling he is out of control, then the situation may be about to get physical. Impending violence is almost certain if the person begins to violate your personal space, makes a fist, or has a flushed face with flaring nostrils.

During these times a fighter can be gentle, but firm. Even though dodging verbal assaults is all about calm responses and treating the other person with dignity, you can do this without behaving like a victim. Behaving like a victim will send the wrong signal to an angry person who is a predator looking for prey.

Again, Michael Kuhr is the perfect example. His is the textbook case on how to de-escalate a situation. He was firm but gentle. He didn't back down from a loudmouth but kindly redirected the man's anger. He didn't act frightened. He simply remained calm, used a bit of humor to distract the man, and actually empathized with the angry patron. He also allowed the man a way out to save face.

It often isn't what you say but how you say it and the tone with which you say it. Asking questions to better understand a situation is sometimes helpful. You cannot completely control the other person's anger, but you can control how you react.

As long as the person is complying with what you need him or her to do, it really doesn't matter what the verbal attacker says. The exception is when the words the person is using are simply inflaming more violence, such as serving to elevate the attacker's own anger or motivating any companions to become a problem.

Pay more attention to the person's behavior. Body language will reveal more during rage than attitude.

Utilize the technique of expressing that you know how they feel. You've felt the same way or you understand. Then redirect if necessary.

"Let me make sure I understand what you're saying" is a good phrase. Then paraphrasing what they just said in a calm manner. Michael Kuhr did this. When the loudmouth spouted off a profanity about Kuhr's mother, Kuhr acknowledged he heard him by saying he could not do those things to his mother. She was too old for him. He politely and humorously addressed the man's words.

While you can treat everyone with respect, remain calm, watch behavior, and speak softly to an angry person, it doesn't work with everyone and the same responses don't work with everyone. Perhaps with the exception of, "Let me make sure I understand." That phrase is pretty safe for the most part.

In 1972, astronaut Neil Armstrong was in Japan speaking to schoolchildren about his experience on the moon. There is a story about a young girl who asked Armstrong what was the moon really like.

Trying to insert humor, Armstrong replied that he didn't find a man in the moon or any green cheese. The Japanese translator told the children that Armstrong had said; "I didn't find any rabbits on the moon." It was actually a good translation.[9]

Western culture talks about a man in the moon or the moon being made of cheese as folklore. But in Eastern cultures there are no such stories about a man in the moon or green cheese. Eastern folklore sees a rabbit in the moon.

So although the words are different, the meaning is the same when the translator relayed Armstrong's humor. The point is that how you respond to one person may be different from how you respond to another. It depends on their background, culture, situation, and even educational level. Each person understands meaning differently.

Angry people also rarely mean what they say. Just because they say they are going to do some terrible thing doesn't mean they will actually follow through. But again, watch their behavior and understand if chemicals or rage fuels the words.

Dr. George Thompson was an English professor who became a police officer and black belt. Before his death in 2011, Dr. Thompson popularized a program called Verbal Judo. He taught police how to communicate effectively.

Dr. Thompson related a story in which someone was holding hostages during his tenure as a police officer. The hostage taker said he would like a million dollars and a plane. As the negotiator, Dr. Thompson humorously responded, "So would I."

He then went on to tell the guy that all those police officers with guns outside weren't going to allow that to happen. But he could work with the guy and make sure the guy lived and not get into deeper trouble. In other words, he didn't lie to the hostage taker. He simply built a rapport and focused on what they could do together.

Through the Verbal Judo Institute, Dr. Thompson taught five universal truths:

1. People want to be respected.
2. People would rather be asked than told.
3. People want to know why.
4. People prefer options rather than threats.
5. People want a second chance.

VICTORY WITHOUT VIOLENCE

In almost every karate class around the world, the common lesson is that martial arts should only be used for self-defense. Martial artists should avoid violence. But seldom are there martial artists like Dr. Thompson who taught verbal martial arts or Michael Kuhr who practices it.

There is a martial artist who gave a demonstration promising to reveal the most effective technique to defend against robbery at gunpoint. He then had an assistant point a training gun at him and inform him that this was a robbery.

The martial artist then said to the class he was about to demonstrate the most effective technique against this and many other violent confrontations. He then turned and ran as fast as he could away from the potential robber.

Now this obviously wouldn't work in every situation. Especially, if a loved one was with you with whom you needed to protect or if there is no way to escape. But it's an important lesson. Quickly running away has merit. Studies have shown that whether someone runs in a straight line or zigzag pattern as recommended by some experts, the runner has about a 50 percent chance of not getting hit by the gunman while running away.[10] The idea is to get out of the line of aim of the gun. Then run quickly.

A confrontation with a gun or robbery is a clear act of violence. In most other situations, words are the first weapon that is utilized. De-escalation is the key to victory over violence in nonphysical violent situations until the situation is calm or you can separate yourself from the confrontation and walk away. It is the same concept as running from a gunman, but you have to find an opening to get away or it may be a situation from which you can't walk away. How you wield words may be the first weapon you use to defend yourself.

Typically, if you respond to violent words in a manner that threatens the aggressor, challenges him, or appears disrespectful the situation will only escalate. Doing the opposite wins the war on words. Use words that are nonthreatening, compromise rather than challenge, and are respectful.

Understand that the intent of the aggressor or the aggressor's cognitive understanding will determine if de-escalation is successful. Someone who is intent on a fight may escalate violence regardless of what is said in response. The aggressor may be simply looking for justification.

Then there are many with cognitive or social impairments. Alcohol fuels much violence as well. Those with mental conditions such as anti-social personality disorders may pose a real threat and not respond as well to de-escalation efforts, which would make such efforts futile. Each situation and person is different.

Keeping a safe distance, you can first try to use words instead of weapons or fists. Asking questions may work before challenging the aggressor, as patience with the aggressor is vital to de-escalation rather than plunging into physical violence.

VERBAL WAR

Sometimes words are not a precursor to violence. The words are the intended violence and the verbal attacker not only rejects de-escalation efforts but welcomes any verbal attention that is received. In these instances, words are the weapons and the war is simply one over words or ideas.

Words are how we communicate ideas. They are the vehicles utilized to influence others, so our communication should be strategic. Wars of words must be understood as they are waged all around us daily.

The basic foundation of verbal war is that one side wishes to establish its point of view as the correct perspective. There are many methods to accomplish this superiority of perspective. If they appeal to logical debate and rational discourse then it is a reasonable discussion in a search for truth.

But if the opponent instead simply uses words as weapons to push their perspective, then it is a verbal war and civil debate has ended. It is when participants talk past each other. Persuading is not a goal or an option as each has entrenched views. The war is simply for onlookers or to boost morale of supporters with the same view. It makes them feel good to verbally attack those with whom they disagree. The danger is whether this will incite violence among those who are prone to violence or suffer from mental illness. The warrior is less concerned with the sides waging these word wars than with ensuring peace in the end. That is the true goal of the warrior.

These are the times when words become the violence, wishing to destroy an opponent with words. Understand the difference because if the weapons are the words then the user of those words isn't going to be as responsive to typical de-escalation techniques. Understand this is on the global level rather than the personal level. Verbal conflict is nearly always personal. Verbal war is much broader.

The opponent might try to destroy credibility to advance a perspective or strike out in anger toward anyone with an opposing thought. The opposition wishes only their perspective to be heard or viewed as having value. The problem is action follows words. Lives have been lost when people are verbally punished for their views. The punishment soon escalates as more join the fray. It is a dangerous recipe.

It is in these instances that it is necessary to redirect the opponent's energy or words in the same manner as an aikido stylist utilizes an opponent's energy favorably by redirecting it. Rather than engaging in a word fight on the opponent's premise or grounds, the premise must be redirected away from the opponent's perspective. It must be reframed on your terms if you wish to redirect the person in an attempt to engage in rational discourse.

We've discussed weapons quite a bit. There are verbal wars over gun control with both sides simply talking past each other, so that's a good example.

Gun control advocates will frame their argument for more gun control around the gun itself. They add emotion by pushing a gun control agenda when emotions are high after a shooting tragedy. It is a useful method.

Defenders of the Second Amendment respond by reframing the debate on the other causes of human violence such as mental health issues rather than the tools that commit violence. In fact, pointing out that guns are supposed to kill, as that is what they are designed to do, helps prevent being put on the defensive and is an example of reframing the argument. This method is sometimes useful as well.

The reason the gun control advocate is able to make a strong argument is because people are moved more by emotional approaches than fact-based approaches. The heart overcomes the brain in these word wars.

Rather than being defensive in responding to gun control advocates on their terms, reframing allows Second Amendment advocates the opportunity to frame the debate on their terms.

Emotions drive much of human behavior. The reframing can remain on the same emotional basis but appeal to how guns protect the innocent against criminals. For example, if guns are banned, only the lawless will have guns and no one will be able to defend themselves. Without guns a mother alone at home cannot protect her children. This appeals to emotion while still using fact without using the frame of the opponent.

This is an example of how the debate is controlled by whoever controls the framing of the debate. Framing is the perspective through which the verbal debate is viewed. If you do not control the frame or perspective, then you will simply be on defense against the onslaught of accusations. Control the context of the debate and how it is framed rather than simply reacting to word attacks.

The use of words as weapons is simply a way to silence opposing ideas instead of debating them. But the problem with verbal war is that initially it seems to be only a war of words, but it can be designed to eventually escalate.

Shouting, intimidation, bullying, mudslinging, and name-calling are designed to prevent an opposing side from receiving a hearing of their views. Attempts to silence contrary opinion are on the rise from many diverse groups around the world.

George Orwell noted the tendency of elastic language in his 1946 essay, "Politics and the English Language." It wasn't an essay about left- or right-wing politics. It was a chastisement of both and was well stated.

Orwell wrote that, "Political language . . . from conservatives to anarchists . . . is designed to make lies sound truthful and murder respectable and to give an appearance of solidity to pure wind."[11] Orwell recommends we clean up our language and make it clearer rather than using old useless phrases, and understand what we are saying. It won't turn wars of words around immediately, but whoever stops using hostile words first and becomes clearer will ultimately win.

This is a problem in our use of language and certain words without agreeing on the meaning of the words. Orwell would not be surprised with modern day wars with words, and his admonishment to be clearer with language and understanding what we are saying is ever more valid.

Name-calling for the sake of name-calling is a method used to invalidate others by labeling them. But again, the problem is whether this eventually escalates to violence or provokes the mentally unstable.

Harmful words are not new. What is new is calling words themselves a violent act to justify physical violence or retribution against opposing views. This occurs on both sides of the political spectrum as no side is immune and all sides of political discourse have unstable individuals.

Evangelist Rick Warren put it into context best. Our culture has accepted two huge lies. The first is that if you disagree with someone then you must fear or hate them. The second is that to love someone means you agree with everything they believe or do. Both ideas are nonsense.

Warriors can restore rationality and statesmanship when wars of words begin by rising above the war that is fueled by different sides talking past one another. Warriors should be the ones to remain calm and redirect those engaging in word wars the way they might redirect an angry person.

Acknowledge the opposing view. Restate valid points. Find common agreement. Seek solutions without language designed simply to inflame, destroy, or label. It is difficult but starts with one person at a time laying down their weapons of words and becoming clearer with language. Word fights should be over policy rather than being personal. We must understand the words and how to manage the conflict they cause. Specifically, being clear about solutions that can be reached together rather than attacking the wind. It's what people really desire.

Researching Sun Tzu to Orwell reveals the only thing a warrior can truly change is his own habits. Changing ourselves will restore a warrior code or at least preserve it. Honor, integrity, and character begin with the warrior first.

A warrior should remain unaffected and calm as word wars are waged around him, just like Samurai were unaffected by the rain. Looking through the storm of words for common agreement and foundational truth is key to resolving conflict.

We cover verbal war because it's a war with no end and comes from so many sources. It has few solutions. But fighters will be immersed in it periodically and therefore must understand the tactics involved.

RESOLVING VERBAL WAR

A verbal debate isn't won unless the other side agrees you've won or a third party declares a winner. You alone do not decide the fight. It is why fighting with words is so difficult. It is a different construct that ancient masters could not have imagined.

We've seen this isn't a book about individual technique. It is about broader principles. Engaging in a back-and-forth war of words should only have the two methods of winning in mind when engaged. The first is to win over opponents so they will acknowledge you are the winner or to have such a strong argument that the third party will declare you are the winner and reward you with whatever the bounty of the argument may be, whether it is votes or some other prize.

Both those methods will not work unless the other side or the third party is respected, is asked rather than told, understands why, is given options rather than threats, and is given a way out or a second chance. It is Thompson's verbal judo on a global scale or Michael Kuhr diffusing a situation. Opposing sides yelling at each other just creates noise, doesn't persuade the opposition, and only annoys the third party you are trying to influence. And no one can resolve this conflict without talking rationally and amicably to someone with whom they disagree.

There is a third method to win as well. It is finding common ground and starting from there. This requires statesmanship, and a politician isn't necessarily a statesman any more than a fighter is automatically a warrior. There is a difference.

Politicians have destroyed the culture of the Samurai by their corruption. But a statesman makes decisions based on principle guided by a moral compass such as a warrior code. A statesman is able to articulate a vision in clear language devoid of inflaming words and can build a consensus to achieve a mutually beneficial vision.

Samurai means to serve. Statesmen should serve as well and could be the new Samurai if they were to look beyond themselves at something greater. Principles of statesmanship and honor are what will win the war on words.

Words are the first weapons drawn in battle. Warriors must learn to wield them carefully.

Notes

1. John Sumser, *A Guide to Empirical Research in Communication* (Thousand Oaks, CA: SAGE Publications, 2001).
2. Yamamoto Tsunetomo, *The Hagakure* (New York: Kodansha International, 1983).
3. "About Maimonides," *Daily Quoted Blog*, http://www.dailyquoted.com/users/maimonides.
4. George Thompson and Jerry Jenkins, *Verbal Judo* (New York: William Morrow & Company, 2013).
5. Kate Lombardi, "Verbal Persuasion for Police," *New York Times*, March 19, 1995.
6. Justin Gammill, "The 4 Stages of Life According to Carl Jung," *Iheartintelligence.com*, October 28, 2015, http://iheartintelligence.com/2015/10/28/carl-jung/.
7. Michael Kuhr, *Kuhr Security*, n.d., http://www.kuhr-security.de/en/.
8. Judo Guy, "Bouncer Kickbox World Champion vs Loudmouth," August 20, 2015, https://www.youtube.com/watch?v=58of-AAHsqM.
9. Ellen Dowling, *The Standup Trainer* (Lincoln, NE: iUniverse, 2000).
10. Greg Ellifritz, "Don't Run in a Straight Line," *Activeresponsetraining.net*, July 11, 2013, http://www.activeresponsetraining.net/dont-run-in-a-straight-line-and-other-bad-advice.
11. George Orwell [1946], "Politics and the English Language," http://www.orwell.ru/library/essays/politics/english/e_polit/.

INDEX

INDEX

INDEX

gun fu, 120
Gunsite Academy, 77

Hadrian, Emperor, 118
Hagakure, The (Yamamoto Tsunetomo), 46–47, 220
Hetherington, Tim, 110
Hick-Hyman Law, 146
Hillaker, Harry, 144
Hombu dojo, 71
honor, 125, 169, 191–201, 233
 character, 164, 166–167
 Commando Kelly, 56
 groups, 123–124, 168
 Kuhr on, 225
 military, 158
 moral codes, 11–12
 Rudy, 97
 Samurai, 83
 war of words, 235
Horne, Patrick Van, 35

I-Ching, 68
Iliad, The (Homer), 193
Inazo Nitobe, 194
Integrity, 88, 193, 195, 198, 200, 224, 233
In the Gravest Extreme (Ayoob), 25
"Invisible Gorilla" study, 22
irrational belief, 154
Israel Defense Forces, 122
Iyengar, Sheena, 146–147

Jastrow, Robert, 100
Jenkins, Jerry, 223
Jinn, Qui-gonn (*Star Wars* character), 109
John Wick (film), 120–121, 126, 128, 167
Joint Special Operations Command, 69
Jordan, Michael, 156
judo, 2, 123, 175, 220, 222
 verbal judo, 223, 228, 234
jujutsu, 123, 127, 220
 ketsugo do, 127, 237
Jung, Carl, 223
Junger, Sebastian, 110

Kamen, Robert Mark, 43
karambit, 208
Karate Kid, The (film), 43
Keller, Gary, 72
Kelly, Charles "Commando," 56
ketsugo do jujutsu, 127, 237
Khan, Genghis, 121–122
kiai, 106
kinetic linking, 88–90, 93–94, 105, 181
King, Stephen, 104
King of Wu, 42–43
King Solomon, 1, 191
knife, 36, 106, 123, 136, 207, 211, 215
 common carry, 206
 range, 208
 speed, 212
knights, 124, 196, 201
Korengal Valley, 110
krav maga, 122, 211

Kuhr, Michael, 224–227, 229, 234
Kung Fu, 99
Kyokushin karate, 87

Lao Tzu, 170
law of reciprocity, 98
Leach, John, 80
LEAPS, 223
Leatham, Rob, 214–215
Lee, Bruce, 4, 27, 88–90, 107–108, 208
 efficiency, 67, 72
 Enter the Dragon, 15
 focus, 104
 Long Beach, 87
 size, 48
 speed, 92–94, 181
Lepper, Mark, 146–147
lethality, 54, 57–64, 165, 177, 208
 aggression, 55, 176, 183
 defined, 53
 General McChrystal on, 70
Lewis, Joe, 125
Lincoln, Abraham, 118
Locke, John, 209
Long Beach International Karate Championships, 87
Longstreet (TV program), 107
Lord Naoshige, 46
Lott, John, 61–62
Lovette, Ed, 25
loyalty, 192, 195, 198
lust, 4

Magellan, Ferdinand, 123
Maimon, Rabbi Moshe ben, 220
Malaysia, 122–123
Mandela, Nelson, 5
Maori, 124
Mao Tse-tung, 92
Marcaida, Doug, 208
Marine Corps Martial Arts Program, 122
Marshall, S. L. A., 56
Martin, Frank, 2
Mastering Karate (Oyama), 87
Master Ummon, 81
Masutatsu Oyama, 87–90
Mattis, James, 178–179, 201
Mayweather, Floyd, Jr., 90
McAuliffe, Anthony, 158
McChrystal, Stanley A., 69–70
McRaven, William, 83, 159–160
Meiji Restoration, 196
Mella, Alberto, 18
militia, 209–210
Miller, Johnny, 9, 16, 31–32, 44, 127
mindfulness, 98
mind-set, 13–14, 21, 46, 49, 59, 64, 107, 117, 219, 223
 combat, 213–214
Ming dynasty, 122
Mings, 122
Miyamoto Musashi (Samurai), 14, 48, 53, 67, 77, 107
MMA, 48, 119

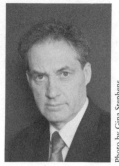

ABOUT THE AUTHOR

PHILLIP STEPHENS is a fifth-degree black belt in Ketsugo Do jujutsu. He won the world championship in the self-defense division at the 2002 Sport Karate Amateur International (SKIL) World Championships held in Panama City, Florida. He was the silver medalist in the National Black-belt League (NBL) self-defense division during the 2003 World Championships held in Houston, Texas, after a perfect season of 10 first-place wins on the East Coast. He also holds numerous regional and state titles, all in the self-defense divisions of martial arts tournaments sanctioned by the Martial Arts Tournament Tour, SKIL, and NBL organizations.

In 2013, Stephens was appointed to the North Carolina Boxing Commission, which regulates combat sports, including boxing and mixed martial arts, where he serves as a commissioner. One of the first chairmen of this commission was former boxing heavyweight world champion James "Bonecrusher" Smith.

Stephens has a doctorate of health science and has practiced emergency medicine as a physician assistant since 1990. He has served as an adjunct faculty member at several medical schools, including A. T. Still University, where he has taught topics such as research methodology and evidence-based medicine.

Married with two children, he enjoys writing in many genres and has other publications, including "The Inside Edge: Emergency Medicine," (ISBN 978-1496-38602-1) a medical textbook published by Wolters Kluwer in 2018. He still volunteers time at a local martial arts dojo owned by fellow martial artists who share his passion for the combative arts.

ABOUT THE ILLUSTRATOR

ROGER MUSASHI REEDER was born in the city of Ritto, which is located in the Shiga prefecture of Japan. His mother is Japanese and his father is American.

He learned calligraphy as part of his Japanese education. Curious about his American heritage, he attended college and grad school in the United States, where he currently works as an emergency medicine pharmacist.

He holds a first degree Black Belt in Shorinji-kempo.

ABOUT THE FOREWORD AUTHOR

The author of some twenty books and thousands of articles relating to self-defense, MASSAD AYOOB has been a firearms and deadly force instructor for 45 years, a police officer for 43, and an expert witness in weapons and homicide cases for 38. He has been ranked as a master instructor in defensive tactics (police unarmed combat and restraint), and was the first five-gun master in the International Defensive Pistol Association.

BOOKS FROM YMAA

DVDS FROM YMAA

more products available from . . .
YMAA Publication Center, Inc. 楊氏東方文化出版中心
1-800-669-8892 • info@ymaa.com • www.ymaa.com